MOBILE INTEGRATED HEALTHCARE

Approach to Implementation

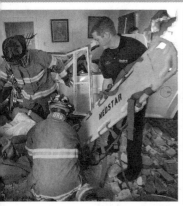

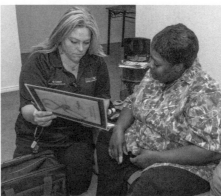
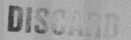
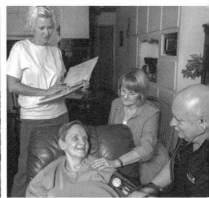

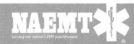

NAEMT

Matt Zavadsky, MS-HSA, EMT

Director of Healthcare and Community Integration

MedStar Mobile Healthcare

Fort Worth, Texas

Douglas Hooten, MBA

Executive Director

MedStar Mobile Healthcare

Fort Worth, Texas

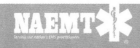

MOBILE INTEGRATED HEALTHCARE

Approach to Implementation

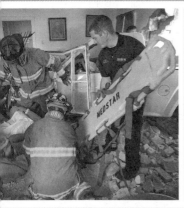
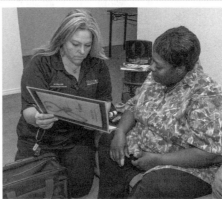
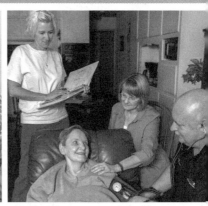

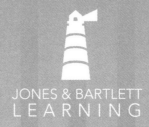

JONES & BARTLETT
LEARNING

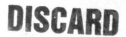

World Headquarters
Jones & Bartlett Learning
5 Wall Street
Burlington, MA 01803
978-443-5000
info@jblearning.com
www.jblearning.com

Jones & Bartlett Learning books and products are available through most bookstores and online booksellers. To contact Jones & Bartlett Learning directly, call 800-832-0034, fax 978-443-8000, or visit our website, www.jblearning.com.

Production Credits

Chief Executive Officer: Ty Field
President: James Homer
Chief Product Officer: Eduardo Moura
VP, Executive Publisher: Kimberly Brophy
Executive Editor—EMS: Christine Emerton
Senior Editor: Barbara Scotese
Production Editor: Jessica deMartin
VP, Sales—Public Safety Group: Matthew Maniscalco
Director of Sales, Public Safety Group: Patricia Einstein
VP, Marketing: Alisha Weisman

VP, Manufacturing and Inventory Control: Therese Connell
Art Development Editor: Joanna Lundeen
Composition: diacriTech
Cover and Text Design: Scott Moden
Manager of Photo Research, Rights, and Permissions: Lauren Miller
Cover Image: Left photo: © Glen E. Ellman; middle and right photos: © Bob Strickland Photography
Printing and Binding: Edwards Brothers Malloy
Cover Printing: Edwards Brothers Malloy

Library of Congress Cataloging-in-Publication Data
Mobile integrated healthcare : approach to implementation / MedStar Mobile Healthcare.
  p. ; cm.
Includes bibliographical references and index.
ISBN 978-1-4496-9016-8
I. MedStar Mobile Healthcare, issuing body.
[DNLM: 1. Mobile Health Units—organization & administration. 2. Delivery of Health Care, Integrated—organization & administration. 3. Emergency Medical Services—organization & administration. WX 190]
R858
610.285—dc23
                                        2014029339

6048

Printed in the United States of America
18 17 16 15 14   10 9 8 7 6 5 4 3 2 1

To all EMS innovators who are changing the way we deliver healthcare to our communities, and of course, to Tessa and Jan, our wives, who have put up with our passion and schedules for years!

Contents

Contributors

Sean Burton, EMT-P, CCEMTP
Clinical Programs Manager
MedStar Mobile Healthcare
Fort Worth, Texas

Maureen Bisognano
President/CEO
Institute for Healthcare Improvement
Cambridge, Massachusetts

J. Daniel Bruce, LCSW, CCM, GCM
Administrator
Klarus Home Care
Fort Worth, Texas

Monica Cushion
Director of Market Development
VITAS Healthcare
Fort Worth, Texas

Steven Q. Davis, MD, MS, LP
Interim/Associate Medical Director
MedStar Mobile Healthcare
Fort Worth, Texas

Larry Erickson
Mobile Integrated Healthcare Client

Antoine Hall
Mobile Integrated Healthcare Client

Rahul Rastogi, MS, MD
Director of Operations for
    Continuing Care Services and
    Quality Value Management
Kaiser Permanente
Northwest Permanente, PC, Physicians &
    Surgeons
Clackamas, Oregon

David Williams, PhD
Chief Executive
Medic Health
Austin, Texas

Dawn Zieger
Project Director – Community Health
John Peter Smith Health Network
Fort Worth, Texas

Reviewers

Debra L. Bell, MS, NREMT-P
Atlanticare Regional Medical Center EMS
  & Inspira Health Network EMS
Atlantic City, New Jersey

Stephen Blackburn, AAS, EMT-P
Lenoir Community College
Kinston, North Carolina

Elliot Carhart, EdD, RRT, NRP
Jefferson College of Health Sciences
Roanoke, Virginia

Keith Carter, BS, NRP, CCP, LP, FP-C
Pafford EMS/Air One
Ruston, Louisiana

Frederick Fowler, EMT-P
Wilton EMS
Saratoga Springs, New York

Michael Hall, MBA, NREMT-P
Nature Coast EMS
Lecanto, Florida

Keith Noble, MS, LP
Austin/Travis City EMS
Austin, Texas

Mark Rector, NREMT-P
Priority Dispatch, Inc.
Salt Lake City, Utah

Matthew Short, LP
BRMC EMS
Texas Tech University Health Sciences
  Center
Lubbock, Texas

Sara VanDusseldorp, NRCCEMTP, NCEE
North Lake County EMS
Waukegan, Illinois

Foreword

In my plenary address at the IHI National Forum on Quality Improvement in Health Care (December 2013), I urged healthcare leaders and caregivers to "flip health care." Those of us focused on improving health and health care for everyone, everywhere, need to build on the models proving so successful in education today. "Flipping the classroom" has been shown to produce much better results, especially for those children most in need. In flipped classrooms, the teachers have the students watch the lectures at home or in the library on video, and then use classroom time for working together and learning actively. The results are great for kids, and the teachers have a better chance of identifying those needing more help in these active classrooms. The teachers also find that they love this new method…moving from what Alison King called the "sage on the stage to the guide on the side." Virtually every sector of the healthcare industry needs this kind of 180-degree change in thinking. Old approaches aren't working. Incremental change doesn't move fast enough. We need more innovation, now.

This book flips emergency care in a beautiful way! Mobile integrated healthcare is an innovative and patient-centered approach to meeting the needs of patients and their families. The model does require you to flip your thinking about almost everything—from the roles of healthcare providers, to what an EMT or paramedic might do to care for a patient in their home, to how the care will get paid for in the future.

The authors teach us how to flip our thinking about using home visits to assess safety and health. They encourage new ways to relate to and support these patients. They urge us to use *all* of the assets in a community to provide better care. This is our shared professional challenge, and it will take new models, new relationships, and new skills.

It goes beyond emergency care. We need innovation in this field to strengthen all of healthcare. Seeing the whole of the patient's needs and assets will be the key to thriving in this new era of healthcare reform and accountable care. To achieve the Institute for Healthcare Improvement Triple Aim, we'll need to integrate care in new ways to improve the health of the population, to improve the experience of care, and to reduce per capita costs.

Making these changes does mean we need new ways to see. And as the new medical school launched by Hofstra University and North Shore-Long Island Jewish is showing, seeing the whole of the patient's life is a key lever for improving care and outcomes. At the new school, medical students begin their education in the field. The first months of medical school are devoted to becoming certified EMTs, and the first patients the students ever see, are seen in their homes or at their workplaces. This is flipping how these medical students understand the real lives of patients. This is flipping their view on how to care for these patients, and it's expanding the vision of the needs and resources available to help them.

And so we all need new ways to see—to see what patients need and what assets they and their family bring, to see across the traditional boundaries of the health care system, and to see new ways that others in the community might come together to provide safe and effective care both during emergencies and throughout the year. The authors prompt us to begin this journey by assessing and understanding local context. They then prompt us to act with practical tools, as well as sharing examples and ideas to get started on innovation and improvement journeys. The message is clear: we have amazing and untapped potential in our communities. And with a deep understanding of community organizing and quality improvement, together we can make a big step forward to the Triple Aim.

As I work with health systems from Sweden to New Zealand, from Malawi to New Orleans, I am seeing an amazing shift in some communities. Now I'll often hear a physician, EMT, nurse, or pharmacist answer the question "what do you do?" in a new way. Some will say "I have two jobs; the first is an EMT and the second is to make the work better." They now see *improvement* as their second job. This commitment to improvement not only fulfills our professional obligations to make care better, it also adds joy to our work. If you visit IHI in Cambridge, Massachusetts, and I do hope you will, you'll see an old Irish adage on the wall. It says "When you come upon a wall, throw your hat over it, and then go get your hat." That's what this book does. It looks over the walls to the potential we need to build for all the patients in our communities, and boldly throws its hat over. So, enjoy this book, and go get your hats!

Maureen Bisognano
President and CEO
Institute for Healthcare Improvement
www.ihi.org
February 2014

1

The Current State of Healthcare and the EMS System

It's a pivotal time in the healthcare system of the United States. Over the last 2 decades, healthcare costs have spiraled out of control. Despite a level of healthcare expenditures that would have seemed unthinkable a generation ago, the health of the population in the United States has improved only marginally. Compared with other economically developed countries, the health status and life expectancy of the U.S. population have actually declined.

Healthcare Expenditures

In 2011 the United States per capita healthcare expenditures (which are the sum of public and private health expenditures, divided by the population) were $8,608, with an average life expectancy of 79 years (**Figure 1-1**). This compares to per capita spending of $3,609 in the United Kingdom, $4,952 in France, and $4,875 in Germany. In fact, most of the European Union spends less than $5,000 per capita on healthcare,[1] with an average life expectancy of 80 years. The United States spends two and a half times the Organisation for Economic Co-operation and Development (OECD) average. Generally, U.S. citizens lag behind in virtually every health statistic measured, including rates of obesity, infant mortality, and preventable illnesses such as diabetes (**Figures 1-2** through **1-5**). Obesity rates have increased substantially during the past 20 years and are highest in the United States. Some experts have predicted that if the current pace of expenditure growth continues, costs could reach $13,330 per capita by 2030, consuming 28% of total national gross domestic product (the market value of all goods and services produced in a country in a given year).[2]

The OECD provides a forum in which governments can work together to share experiences and seek solutions to common problems. The organization works with governments to understand what drives economic, social, and environmental change. The OECD forum measures productivity and global flows of trade and investment and analyzes and compares data to predict future trends.

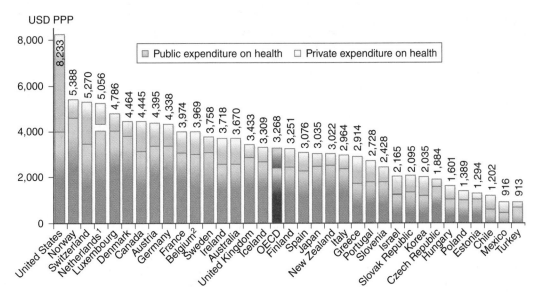

Figure 1-1 International comparison of health expenditures; the total health expenditure per capita, public and private, 2010 (or nearest year).

1. In the Netherlands, it is not possible to clearly distinguish the public and private share related to investments.
2. Total expenditure excluding investments.

Data from: Organisation for Economic Co-operation and Development.

Causes of High Costs

Experts credit the largely quantity-based payment system in the United States as the primary reason why healthcare costs are escalating. Healthcare providers are not given incentives to help patients navigate the healthcare system or keep them healthy. Instead, healthcare providers are rewarded financially by the number of billable procedures they perform as a primary source of revenue. The more patient procedures that are performed, the higher the revenues for the providers. Providers therefore have incentives to schedule visits and procedures.

Hospitals market services to attract patients to increase revenue. Drive along any highway in America and you will see billboards from hospitals that advertise everything from short waits in their emergency department to their excellence in cardiac care. When the number of patient procedures performed and the cost of those procedures are considered, it is clear why the United States healthcare system expenditures outpace every other country (**Tables 1-1** and **1-2**).

The Impact of Healthcare Costs on the World of EMS

The revenue structure of the emergency medical services (EMS) system is no different than that of doctors and hospitals. Medicare, Medicaid, and subsequently most commercial insurers recognize

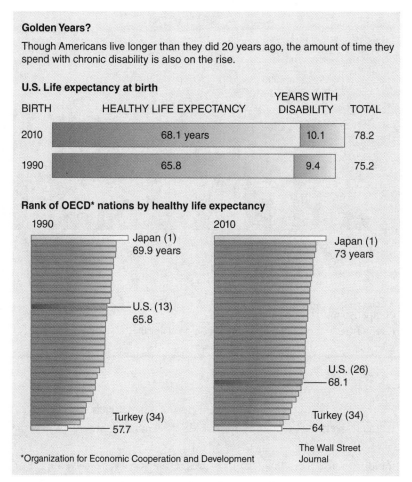

Figure 1-2 Healthy life expectancy, international comparison.
Data from: Institute for Health Metrics and Evaluation, Seattle.

emergency medical transportation as a benefit and therefore billable under health insurance plans. EMS providers have a revenue incentive to transport patients.

Historically, an EMS business development strategy has largely centered around increasing the number of patients transported to the hospital emergency department rather than taking steps to help patients navigate the healthcare system to ensure that they are provided the best, most appropriate resources for their care. The EMS system benefits financially from patients using one of the most expensive transportation resources, an ambulance, to deliver them to one of the most expensive settings for healthcare, an emergency department (ED). Hospital and ED staff have encouraged

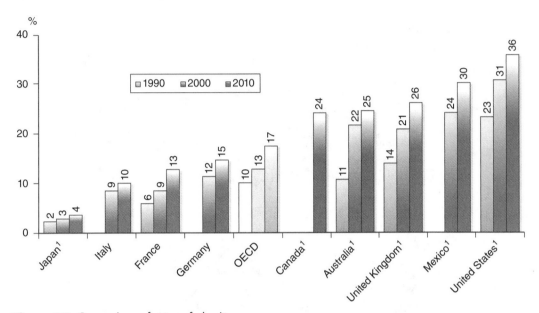

Figure 1-3 Comparison of rates of obesity.
1. Data are based on measurements rather than self-reported height and weight.
Data from: Organisation for Economic Co-operation and Development.

EMS providers to promote transport as the best option for patients who call 9-1-1. This is the traditional "you call, we haul" mentality most EMS systems and providers have been operating under.

The EMS industry also faces financial pressures. Have you ever received a call from a hospital EMS coordinator wondering why you are not transporting more patients to their facility? Does your system have policies requiring you to tell patients, who need to acknowledge they've been told in writing, that if they refuse transport to the ED they could die? Were you ever told that you needed to transport more patients so that the agency could buy new equipment?

Other Factors that Affect Healthcare
The Now Generation
People have become accustomed to getting everything now. A letter sent in the mail is too slow, so email, text messaging, and instantaneous responses and service have become the norm. This expectation is found in all areas of the medical field as well. Why go through painful, long-term physical therapy to correct a knee condition when a knee replacement can be done? Why wait for an

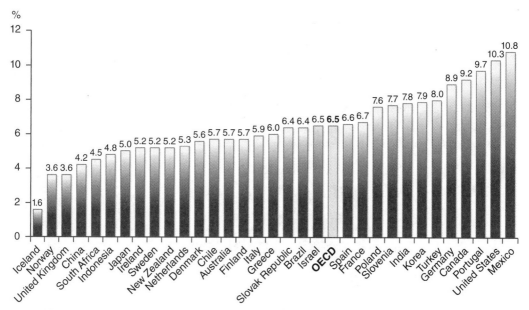

Figure 1-4 Comparison of rates of diabetes. Prevalence estimates of diabetes in adults aged 20–79 years, 2010.

Note: The data cover both type 1 and type 2 diabetes.

Data from: Organisation for Economic Co-operation and Development.

appointment with a primary care physician who knows the patient well and can coordinate care, when a trip to the emergency department will get more immediate results?

The "now" expectation is one of the primary economic drivers behind urgent care clinics (some of which are developing franchises) and the explosion of free-standing emergency departments in urban areas across the United States. It's also one of the primary reasons people call 9-1-1 to access the healthcare system. It's simple, easy, and, in most areas, results in a healthcare provider in the patient's home within 10 minutes.

The Growing Physician Shortage

Hospitals and Health Networks published a report in March 2013 highlighting the predicted physician shortage. The aging baby boomers requiring additional medical care and the predicted surge of insured patients as a result of healthcare finance reform are primarily driving this shortage. There's a growing shortage of physicians that is only expected to get worse after full implementation of the Affordable Care Act. The Association of Medical Colleges anticipates

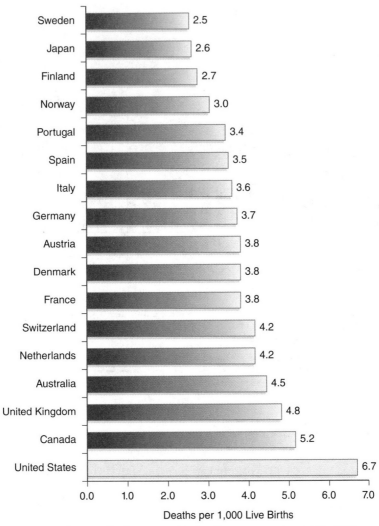

Figure 1-5 Comparison of rates of infant mortality in 17 peer countries, 2005–2009.
Note: Rates were averaged through 2005 to 2009.
Data from: Organisation for Economic Co-operation and Development.

that the shortage in all specialties will grow from 7,400 in 2008 to 130,600 by 2025 (65,000 in primary care alone) (**Figure 1-6**).

Although the scope of practice for EMS providers is restricted, for decades they have been used as physician extenders, serving as the on-scene eyes and ears of the physicians. The mobile integrated healthcare model enhances this physician extension.

Table 1-1 Where the U.S. Health System Does More than Other Countries

	United States	Rank Compared with OECD Countries	OECD Average
MRI units	31.6 per million population	2nd	12.5 per million population
MRI exams	97.7 per 1,000 population	2nd	46.3 per 1,000 population
CT scanners	40.7 per million population	3rd	22.6 per million population
CT exams	265.0 per 1,000 population	3rd	123.8 per 1,000 population
Tonsillectomy	254.4 per 100,000 population	1st	130.1 per 100,000 population
Coronary bypass	79.0 per 100,000 population	3rd	47.3 per 100,000 population
Knee replacements	226.0 per 100,000 population	1st	121.6 per 100,000 population
Caesarean sections	32.9 per 100 live births	6th	26.1 per 100 live births

Note: OECD, Organisation for Economic Co-operation and Development; MRI, magnetic resonance imaging; CT, computed tomography.
Data from: Organisation for Economic Co-operation and Development.

Table 1-2 U.S. Prices for Certain Procedures Are Much Higher than in Other OECD Countries, 2007 U.S. Dollars

Procedures	AUS	CAN	DEU	FIN	FRA	SWE	USA
Appendectomy	5,044	5,004	2,943	3,739	4,558	4,961	7,962
Normal delivery	2,984	2,800	1,789	1,521	2,894	2,591	4,451
Caesarean section	7,092	4,820	3,732	4,808	5,820	6,375	7,449
Coronary angioplasty	7,131	9,277	3,347	5,574	7,027	9,296	14,378
Coronary artery bypass graft	21,698	22,694	14,067	23,468	23,126	21,218	34,358
Hip replacement	15,918	11,983	8,899	10,834	11,162	11,568	17,406
Knee replacement	14,608	9,910	10,011	9,931	12,424	10,348	14,946

Data from: Organisation for Economic Co-operation and Development.

The Broken System

For 30 years the United States has been spending more on healthcare than any other economically developed nation. A positive return on this investment has not been realized in health status or life expectancy. Albert Einstein said that the definition of insanity is doing the same thing over and over while expecting a different outcome. To improve the healthcare of people in the United States, change in the system has to occur.

Currently the U.S. healthcare system is fragmented. Often, patients are not prepared to navigate the system to provide for their own healthcare needs, and the myriad of healthcare providers in the

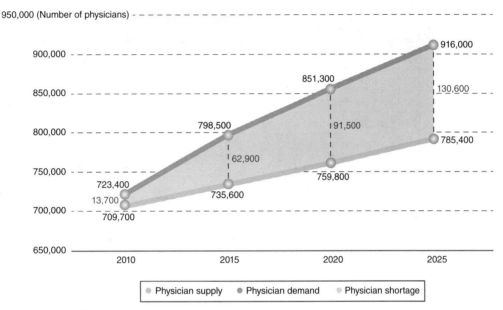

Figure 1-6 The physician gap.
Data from: American Medical Colleges.

system are given financial incentives to do more *to* the patient, not more *for* the patient. A well-developed mechanism for quality care coordination between EMS providers, hospitals, and doctors is not in place. In the current landscape, healthcare is provided by the patient being treated at a healthcare facility, not by providing healthcare in the patient's home. When patients become frustrated with how to navigate this complex system, they often go to the emergency department or call 9-1-1 to access the healthcare system.

In the current broken, overwhelmed healthcare system, people are uneducated about the care available to them so they are forced into using emergency care as their primary source of care. An emergency department is designed to handle episodic emergency events. The emergency department is currently being used to manage a variety of patient issues, including the care of chronic diseases such as diabetes. There is an opportunity now for EMS to be part of the solution as an integral provider within the healthcare delivery system.

The Evolving Role of EMS in Healthcare

For years, EMS providers have considered themselves providers of only emergency care. All levels of training focus on treating acute illnesses and injuries and transporting patients to the hospital emergency department.

John Peter Smith Health Network partnered with MedStar to expand the mobile integrated healthcare program for our patients because we saw first-hand the impact it was having on our patients. As the community's safety net healthcare system, many of our patients have difficulty navigating a very complex healthcare system. Bringing the care to them, where they need it and when they need it, helps us improve patient outcomes and enhance the patient's experience of care with our healthcare system. The paramedics in the field can see things the primary care providers may not see. They can also provide patient-centered education in the patient's home environment, with the patient's family present and part of the educational process. If the patient does call 9-1-1, the mobile healthcare provider can respond to the call and help navigate the patient to the best care setting for their individual healthcare need.

The integration of care across the continuum, from in-patient care to community care using a patient-centered medical home and mobile healthcare resources has had a major impact on 9-1-1, ED and readmission rates for the patients who have been enrolled in this unique partnership between JPS, the patient, and MedStar.

Dawn Zieger
Project Director, Community Health
JPS Health Network

Healthcare reform continually drives changes in the industry, and everyone is struggling to understand where the industry is headed and how EMS providers will need to adapt. What regulatory changes are coming? Will providers be prepared for those changes? The current state of healthcare is not well suited to evaluate the nonclinical needs of a patient in the community. As a result, EMS providers respond to a variety of calls, many of which are not an emergency.

In their 2012 annual report, the National Association of State EMS officials documented that EMS responds to 37 million house calls per year, and 30% of the responses did not result in a patient transport to an emergency department. And, in an analysis done of MedStar's 9-1-1 call volume in 2013, 37% of 9-1-1 calls did not receive a HOT response (**Table 1-3**).

Table 1-3 Percentage Change in Overall Call Volume, 2003–2013

Call Type	% Increase	Call Type	% Decrease
Interfacility	11.32	Psychiatric	3.76
Sick person	10.37	Abdominal pain	2.83
Falls	5.87	Trauma injury	3.71
Unconscious person	5.20	Chest pain	7.97
Assault	4.21	Motor vehicle accident	10.38
Convulsions	4.16	Breathing problems	10.48

Why People Call 9-1-1

People call 9-1-1 because they want to know if they need to go to the hospital. They call to access the healthcare system, they call because it is what they've been taught to do in an emergency, and they call because it's what their doctor's recording tells them to do when they call after hours.

The high rate of low-acuity 9-1-1 calls is partly caused by the current structure of the emergency healthcare system. Patients are conditioned to call 9-1-1 and are often directed to 9-1-1 by other healthcare providers. A voicemail recording at most physician offices says, "If this is an emergency, hang up and call 9-1-1." But what constitutes an emergency? If a parent is worried about his child's escalating fever, stomach pains, or other symptoms, fear increases if he cannot get an appointment with the doctor that day. The alternative is to call 9-1-1 and go to the emergency department. But as mentioned earlier, 37% of the time the situation is not an emergency. Our healthcare system has created and reinforced this process.

Television shows have reinforced the idea that people should call 9-1-1 for any type of problem, and an ambulance and fire department will arrive within a few minutes, with maybe a helicopter shortly thereafter. Often, the depiction of the EMS system on television has given viewers an unrealistic expectation of the care they will receive in the healthcare system.

Regular trips to an emergency department for low-acuity ailments have a negative impact on the overall care the patient receives because typically the care that is given in an emergency department is not coordinated with a patient-centered medical home. In addition, the care of patients in an emergency department uses high-cost resources for conditions that could possibly have been more appropriately managed in a more cost-effective setting.

Mobile Integrated Healthcare Defined

What's in a name? There has been some discussion in the EMS circles about use of the terms *community paramedicine*, or *community paramedic*, versus the term *mobile integrated healthcare*.

The National Association of EMTs convened a workgroup to focus on the transformation of EMS into something else. The workgroup had representation from the following national associations:

- National Association of Emergency Medical Technicians (NAEMT)

- National Association of State EMS Officials (NASEMSO)

- National Association of EMS Physicians (NAEMSP)

- American College of Emergency Physicians (ACEP)

- National EMS Management Association (NEMSMA)

- National Association of EMS Educators (NAEMSE)

- International Academies of Emergency Dispatch (IAED)

- Association of Critical Care Transport (ACCT)

- North Central EMS Institute (NCEMSI)

- Paramedic Foundation

- American Ambulance Association (AAA)

And this group collaborated to define mobile integrated healthcare. The consensus of the group, in its simplest definition, was: Mobile integrated healthcare (MIH) is the provision of healthcare using patient-centered, mobile resources in the out-of-hospital environment that are integrated with the entire spectrum of healthcare and social service resources available in the local community. MIH may include, but is not limited to, such services as[3]:

- Providing telephone advice to 9-1-1 callers instead of resource dispatch

- Providing community paramedicine care, chronic disease management, preventive care, or postdischarge follow-up visits

- Transport or referral to a broad spectrum of appropriate care, not just hospital emergency departments.

The consensus of this group was also that to be successful mobile integrated healthcare programs should be:

- Fully integrated—A vital component of the existing healthcare system, with efficient bidirectional sharing of patient health information

- Collaborative—Predicated on meeting a defined need in a local community articulated by local stakeholders and supported by formal community health needs assessments

- Supplemental—Enhancing existing healthcare systems or resources, and filling the resource gaps within the local community

- Data driven—Data are collected and analyzed to develop evidence-based performance measures, research, and benchmarking opportunities.

- Patient-centered—Incorporating a holistic approach focused on the improvement of patient outcomes

- Recognized as the multidisciplinary practice of medicine—Overseen by engaged physicians and other practitioners involved in the MIH program as well as the patient's primary care network/patient-centered medical home, using telemedicine technology when appropriate and feasible

- Team based—Integrating multiple providers, both clinical and nonclinical, in meeting the holistic needs of patients who are either enrolled in or referred to MIH programs

- Educationally appropriate—Including more specialized education of community paramedics and other MIH providers, with the approval of regulators or local stakeholders

- Consistent with the Institute for Healthcare Improvement's (IHI) Triple Aim® philosophy— Improving the patient experience of care; improving the health of populations; and reducing the per capita cost of healthcare. The Institute for Healthcare Improvement (IHI) is an independent, not-for-profit organization based in Cambridge, Massachusetts. They are a leading innovator, convener, partner, and driver of results in healthcare and healthcare improvement worldwide.

- Financially sustainable—Including proactive discussion and financial planning with federal payers, health systems, accountable care organizations, managed care organizations, physician hospital organizations, legislatures, and other stakeholders to establish MIH programs and component services as an element of the overall IHI Triple Aim approach

- Legally compliant—Through strong, legislated enablement of MIH component services and programs at the federal, state, and local levels

MIH could incorporate the use of community paramedics. These practitioners may be paramedics provided with additional, specialized training with an expanded role of providing patient navigation services or preventive services designed to avoid unnecessary emergency services use or hospitalization. However, MIH programs may use practitioners other than paramedics in this role. They may use EMTs, registered nurses, nurse practitioners, physician assistants, or even physicians. These programs may also incorporate services that go beyond the point of care services in the field, such as programs based in a 9-1-1 call center that provide callers with healthcare advice from nurses.

For these reasons, the term *mobile integrated healthcare* is used to refer to the services provided, and in many, but not all cases, these services may be provided by community paramedics. Appendix A provides a comprehensive list of U.S. agencies developing their own MIH and community paramedicine programs.

EMS Under Fire

In April 2014, the Centers for Medicare and Medicaid Services (CMS) released charge and payment data for all Medicare Part B providers. The communication from CMS that accompanied the release contained the following notable quotes by Jonathan Blum, CMS Principal Deputy Administrator[4]:

> *In letters to the American Medical Association and Florida Medical Association, the Centers for Medicare & Medicaid Services (CMS) announced our intent today to take another major step forward in making our healthcare system more transparent and accountable.*

> *We plan to provide the public unprecedented access to information about the number and type of healthcare services that individual physicians and certain other healthcare professionals delivered in 2012, and the amount Medicare paid them for those services, beginning not earlier than April 9. Providing consumers with this information will help them make more informed choices about the care they receive.*

With the release of ambulance service payment data, the good news is that the EMS profession is clearly being identified by CMS as a "healthcare service" with "healthcare professionals." This is a major step toward validating that EMS professionals are healthcare providers. Given the incredible opportunities to implement programs that meet the IHI's Triple Aim, which is discussed in the next chapter, this recognition positions the EMS profession as a participant in helping the healthcare industry achieve the Triple Aim goals.

The challenge for the EMS industry now, however, is much like the challenge that has been faced by the EMS system's partners for the past 2 years since CMS started publishing charge and payment data for hospitals—how to understand fully what the numbers mean. The CMS charge and payment data, which is the second release of data this year, continues to portray the profession in a less-than-positive light. The CMS Office of the Inspector General (OIG) released their findings on the ambulance industry on September 24, 2013. In the report,[5] the OIG published statements such as:

- "Since 2002, Medicare Part B payments for ambulance transports have grown at a faster rate than all Medicare Part B payments."

- "From 2002 to 2011, the number of beneficiaries who received ambulance transports increased 34%, although the total number of Medicare fee for service beneficiaries increased just 7%."

- "The number of dialysis-related transports increased 269%."

With EMS as the fastest growing Medicare Part B expense, it makes the profession an easy target for fraud investigators and even payers of our services.

In a December 2013 article in the *New York Times*[6] reporting on the OIG's findings, the EMS industry was challenged with the following statements:

In such a fragmented system, it is hard to know how much high-priced ambulance transport contributes nationally to America's $2.7 trillion healthcare bill.

But Medicare, the insurance program for the elderly, does tabulate its numbers and has become alarmed at its fast-rising expenditures for ambulance rides: nearly $6 billion a year, up from just $2 billion in 2002.

Unfortunately, that was not the only national media story about the fraud and abuse in our profession. *Bloomberg BusinessWeek* reported[7] the dark side of ambulance services with a headline that read "Medicare's $5 Billion Ambulance Tab Signals Area of Abuse" and the following statements:

The patient smoked cigarettes in the passenger seat of the ambulance every week, chatting with the driver while taxpayers foot the $1,000 bill to drive him four blocks for his dialysis treatment.

The U.S. Department of Health and Human Services has identified ambulance service as one of the biggest areas of overuse and abuse in Medicare.

To keep them coming back, Penn Choice ambulance drivers would hand out envelopes with $100 to $400 in cash every month to the passengers, many of whom were poor and unable to work because of their health condition, the government said. Leahy said she hasn't prosecuted any of the patients since all have cooperated with the investigation.

At the core of ambulance service is the question of value. What value is the customer placing on EMS? If payers viewed EMS (ambulance transport) as valuable, the cost of the service would be understood—that's basic economic theory. The reality for the EMS profession, however, is that it has fallen short in demonstrating value to payers. There is a lack of any peer-reviewed, published studies that demonstrate that going to the hospital by ambulance, or providing an EMS first response, improves patient outcomes, improves the patient's experience of care, or reduces the patient's overall healthcare costs. At numerous conventions, conferences, and national presentations on mobile integrated healthcare, EMS professionals couldn't identify such studies when asked.

The payers of our healthcare system are moving toward value-based purchasing (VBP). Hospitals have been under a VBP metric since 2012 when Medicare instituted bonuses or penalties based on the hospital's ability to meet specific clinical and patient experience metrics. Physicians will soon be under a similar economic model starting in 2015. As healthcare providers, EMS needs to prepare for a VBP economic model. Among the many challenges with VBP for EMS will be the determination of outcome metrics to be measured and reported. EMS has not developed standardized metrics for a service delivery model that brings value to the payer. The only real metric in EMS, other than cardiac arrest survival, is response time, which has been proven through peer-reviewed scientific studies to not make a significant difference in patient outcome.

The mission of the EMS profession should be to transform the discussion with our payers away from a fee-for-transport model to a VBP model. The true value the profession can bring to the health-care system most likely includes mobile integrated healthcare strategies that safely navigate patients through the complicated healthcare system to meet the IHI Triple Aim. CMS has funded programs such as the CMMI (Centers for Medicare and Medicaid Innovation) grant at the Regional Emergency Medical Services Authority in Reno, Nevada, and the 1115 Waiver project at MedStar Mobile Health-care in Fort Worth, Texas. CMS is interested in MIH for positive reasons. During a meeting in March 2013 with the Chief Medical Officer for CMS, Patrick Conway, MD, expressed strong support for additional demonstration projects for EMS-based MIH programs in an effort to increase the numbers of patients enrolled in these programs. With a larger patient population, EMS can work together with CMS to shape the EMS payment model of the future.

The University of Pittsburgh Medical Center (UPMC) CONNECT Community Paramedic project in Pittsburgh, Pennsylvania, and the Community Paramedic program with Kaiser and MetroWest Ambulance in Portland, Oregon, have sparked keen interest in the value of MIH with large payer systems such as Highmark Blue Cross and Kaiser. The National Highway Transportation and Safety Administration (NHTSA) recently released a request for proposal to groups to work on a proposed redesign of the future economic model for EMS. The proposals sent back to NHTSA and the Office of the Assistant Secretary of Preparedness and Response will no doubt include ideas for VBP in EMS either with some type of global payment model or outcome-based payment system, regardless of whether or not the patient was transported to the hospital.

Innovation in Healthcare

Something radical must occur to interrupt the current healthcare model, and EMS providers can lead the charge. The solution involves innovation. In 2009 when MedStar started their mobile integrated healthcare program with Tarrant County, Texas, a quick response vehicle (QRV) responded to basic 9-1-1 calls instead of an ambulance. The program identified 21 patients who called 9-1-1 fifteen or more times in 90 days. These patients generated nearly 2,000 9-1-1 calls in 1 year alone. The implementation of the new mobile integrated healthcare model to educate this core group of frequent callers and to connect them with the appropriate healthcare resources resulted in a 78% reduction in 9-1-1 calls or the patients enrolled in the program.

One high-risk patient with heart failure called 9-1-1 forty-three times in 2012 because of congestive heart failure, emphysema, and diabetes. Her conditions made her an ideal candidate for the new program, which would bring healthcare into her home. The patient graduated from the 12-month program in January 2013 with a reduction in the number of ambulance transports to eight.

Mobile integrated healthcare brings healthcare to patients instead of relying on patients to manage their care on their own. The process is centered on prevention, education, and helping patients navigate the healthcare system. It offers individuals in need of a better patient experience onsite treatment for care such as checking vital signs, reviewing medical needs, and education about their medications—all in the comfort of their own homes.

"They come here and check my vital signs," the patient said, "and if there's something wrong, they tell me what to do and how to do it."

The Future of Mobile Integrated Healthcare

MedStar's mobile integrated healthcare program has already saved close to $1 million in healthcare expenditures and has the potential to save millions more. The program also improves patient care by helping patients connect with the resources they need to maintain good health and manage their conditions.

Although EMS personnel have traditionally considered themselves providers of emergency care, the types of calls that providers have been responding to paint a different picture. In the past, 9-1-1 has been a safety net for both emergency and nonemergency care. At MedStar's communications center, an Accredited Center of Excellence, a quality review of 12 months of 9-1-1 requests coming to the call center revealed that 36.6% of the 9-1-1 requests did not get a light and siren response. Meaning, based on the Advanced Medical Priority Dispatch System®, these calls did not need a HOT response or require an emergency medical responder.

On the basis of accurate and dependable information obtained by the emergency medical dispatcher, therefore, more than a third of 9-1-1 calls are not classified as emergencies. Educating the public when *not* to call 9-1-1, however, is not a patient-centered solution. In most cases, the patient is the *least* prepared person to determine whether or not the situation warrants an emergency response. It is far better to continue fielding 9-1-1 calls to determine what type of help is best for the patient. There is no such thing as an inappropriate 9-1-1 *request,* but there is such a thing as an inappropriate *response* to that request.

Under the previous model at MedStar, which still exists in communities all across the nation, patients are transported to the emergency department in the back of an ambulance after they have called 9-1-1. When they are discharged, they are sent home, and without adequate transitional care the cycle is often repeated. These patients are referred to in the industry as "frequent flyers" because they call 9-1-1 frequently and end up in the hospital system when often the situation is not an emergency. Abuse of the healthcare system is costly to payers, hospitals, doctors, and EMS providers, and the lack of care coordination is not optimal for the patient's outcome. Patients need to receive education in a different way to manage their own healthcare.

Think about the following questions.

- What if a patient with a low-acuity 9-1-1 call were redirected to a triage nurse from the moment the call to 9-1-1 was received?

- What if there were a program in place for high-risk, frequent callers that focused on prevention?

- What if a patient who is not eligible for home health care could receive in-home healthcare that would enable self-monitoring of vital signs, heart rate, or blood sugar levels?

- What if a patient who is not eligible for home healthcare could receive education in self-administering medication properly?

- What if the patient were connected to a physician by the dispatch center nurse navigator and by specially trained EMS personnel creating a long-term relationship?

In the mobile integrated healthcare model, patients are educated in managing their own care better at home, and at the same time, their primary care physician and networks of other providers are brought into the process for a truly integrated healthcare approach. The crucial missing link that this model of care provides is the role of EMS in the coordination of care.

Making Mobile Integrated Healthcare Work

The healthcare process can be confusing and frustrating. When a patient enters the doctor's office there is often a long wait and a brief visit. Under the current economic model, a doctor is aiming to treat enough patients in a day to keep the practice financially viable, which is not ideal for building long-term patient relationships.

One way that specially trained nurse navigators in the dispatch center and EMS personnel can provide care in a patient home setting is by facilitating communication between the dispatch nurse navigator, patient, and doctor. Everyone wins. By focusing on prevention, mobile integrated healthcare can reduce costs and better serve individual needs. The doctors and hospitals will benefit from a reduction in preventable readmissions and unnecessary emergency department visits. When a patient is enrolled in a mobile integrated healthcare program, a provider routinely checks on the patient at home. The provider reviews the patient's vital signs, diet, and medications and administers appropriate medical care to the patient. Often, the care can be as simple as reexplaining instructions given to a patient by a doctor to ensure patient understanding.

In the third year of MedStar's mobile integrated healthcare program, the 38 patients enrolled in the high utilizer group had an 86% reduction in 9-1-1 calls. The reduction in emergency department visits and ambulance usage saved Medicaid a total of $820,000 in expenditures. By the fourth year, the enrollment in the program had grown to 184 patients, who continue to demonstrate an average of an 80–85% reduction in 9-1-1 usage. The financial benefit of the program is tangible and measurable. With the right focus and partnerships within the community, this model of providing healthcare can be duplicated.

The time for change is now. Patient-centered healthcare with a reduction of overall costs for the entire industry is the goal. With the passage of the Affordable Care Act, large amounts of funding have been made available for healthcare providers to implement programs that promote the goals of IHI's Triple Aim.

New Emerging Models in Healthcare

The financial incentives that hospitals and doctors have received for treating a high volume of patients and performing large numbers of services are changing. The focus is shifting to payments based on the patient's outcome. It won't be long before EMS agencies are involved in a patient care performance-based payment model, not just the performance of response times. It would be difficult to point to a published, peer-reviewed study that demonstrates that because the patient came to the hospital by ambulance, the patient's outcome was better, except perhaps for patients with a myocardial infarction or stroke.

Through the innovative and successful MedStar mobile integrated healthcare program, education has begun with all of the stakeholders that it is time to do something different. Creating a healthier industry overall is the higher goal, and mobile integrated healthcare brings the black bag back to the patient's home, providing out-of-hospital care, and it is being provided by a new member of the healthcare team.

The services administered by a mobile integrated healthcare provider bridge the gap between the medical needs of the patient and the community, as well as addressing the social issues that prevent full realization of that medical care. For a physician who is unable to address the barriers limiting a patient's access to care, a mobile integrated healthcare program can support this care and remove the barriers to improving the patient's health. For example, a person with congestive heart failure whose condition is exacerbated after walking up three flights of stairs, resulting in rehospitalization, may need assistance finding a first-floor living accommodation. Or a patient who visits the ED frequently for pain medication refills because family members are selling the patient's medications on the street may need a safe to keep medication locked up. Or a patient who does not visit a community clinic because of a fear of taking public transportation may need help in learning how to ride the bus.

Pearls of WISDOM

The *integrated* part of mobile integrated healthcare requires that you have a good understanding of the healthcare environment. To assist you with that, electronic subscriptions to daily news summaries from sources such as *Kaiser Health News, Hospitals and Health Networks, Modern Healthcare,* and *Fierce Healthcare* will help you stay informed on the current happenings in healthcare.

Are You READY?

- Become a student of the changes occurring in the healthcare system.
- Schedule periodic coffee or breakfast meetings with local key healthcare stakeholders to learn what's happening in their world.
- Subscribe to email alerts from sources like *Hospitals and Health Networks, Kaiser Health News,* and *Modern Healthcare.*
- Start making a list of who the stakeholders are in your community who might have an interest in the development of an MIH program. As more ideas come to mind, add to the list.

Summary

The world of healthcare is changing, and EMS providers, dispatch centers, hospitals, doctors, and patients have to change with it. The solution must address and provide education, access, and navigation to appropriate care. It's about the right care at the right time at the right place. One benefit of EMS organizations worldwide is the existence of communication dispatch centers where the initial call for service occurs, an already trained, 24/7 mobile workforce. EMS organizations have the operational structure in place to do so much more than just respond to 9-1-1 calls or transport patients. Who better to lead change?

References

1. The World Bank. Health expenditures per capita (current US$). Available at: http://data .worldbank.org/indicator/SH.XPD.PCAP. Accessed April 23, 2014.

2. Muñoz E, Muñoz W III, Wise L. National and surgical health expenditures, 2005–2025. *Ann Surg.* 2010;251:195–200. Available at: http://www.ncbi.nlm.nih.gov/pubmed/20054269. Accessed April 23, 2014.

3. National Association of Emergency Medical Technicians. Mobile integrated healthcare and community paramedicine. Available at: http://www.naemt.org/MIH-CP/MIH-CP.aspx. Accessed August 22, 2014.

4. Blum J. Historic release of data delivers unprecedented transparency on the medical services physicians provide and how much they are paid. The CMS blog. Available at: http://blog.cms. gov/2014/04/09/historic-release-of-data-delivers-unprecedented-transparency-on-the-medical-services-physicians-provide-and-how-much-they-are-paid/. Accessed May 7, 2014.

5. Office of the Inspector General, U.S. Dept. of Health and Human Services report (OEI-09-12-00350). Utilization of Medicare ambulance transports, 2002–2011. Available at: https://oig.hhs .gov/oei/reports/oei-09-12-00350.asp. Accessed May 20, 2014.

6. Rosenthal E. Think the E.R. is expensive? Look at how much it costs to get there. *The New York Times.* December 4, 2013. Available at: http://www.nytimes.com/2013/12/05/health/think-the-er-was-expensive-look-at-the-ambulance-bill.html?_r=0. Accessed May 7, 2014.

7. Pettypiece S. Medicare's $5 billion ambulance tab signals area of abuse. *Bloomberg Business Week.* April 23, 2014. Available at: http://www.bloomberg.com/news/2014-04-24/medicare-s-5-billion-ambulance-tab-signals-area-of-abuse.html. Accessed May 7, 2014.

2

Healthcare Reform and Mobile Integrated Healthcare Systems

The Patient Protection and Affordable Care Act (PPACA, or ACA) is often referred to as *healthcare* reform, but it may not be as much healthcare reform as much as it is healthcare *finance* reform. The 1,500-page ACA essentially describes a new way of paying for healthcare, not necessarily how it is to be provided. This reform allows providers to come up with innovative ways to deliver health care under the new payment models.

The changes brought about by the Affordable Care Act have opened the door for positive transformation in healthcare, and EMS can play an important role in this new environment. One of the most significant changes brought about by the ACA has been the accountability placed on the healthcare industry, as reflected by the ambitious approach by the Institute for Healthcare Improvement to broaden the role of community-based services.

The Institute for Healthcare Improvement Triple Aim Initiative

The Institute for Healthcare Improvement (IHI) developed the Triple Aim framework that describes an approach to optimizing health system performance.[1] New system designs must be developed to simultaneously achieve the following:

- Improving the patient experience of care (including quality and satisfaction)

- Improving the health of populations

- Reducing the per capita cost of healthcare

Now the goal of healthcare is to provide better care and achieve better outcomes at a reduced cost. Healthcare providers can no longer operate under the payment model based on the quantity of services. The focus has changed and become patient centered—providing the appropriate level and type of care needed as well as measuring patient outcomes and satisfaction.

Almost every funding opportunity announcement for grant applications and other potential financing use the IHI terminology. Hospital CEOs, hospital CFOs, and other healthcare stakeholders refer to the IHI Triple Aim approach as a guide in the projects that are being undertaken. EMS personnel have

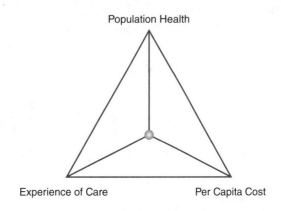

The IHI Triple Aim

Source: IHI Triple Aim. Institute for Healthcare Improvement. http://www.ihi.org/Engage/Initiatives/TripleAim/Pages/default.aspx

to adapt that same philosophy when developing programs. This shift in attitude is the first step toward the acceptance of EMS as a true participant in the improvement of the healthcare system.

EMS as a Healthcare Benefit

Until now, the care provided by the EMS system has been classified by most payers as only a transportation benefit, not a healthcare benefit. As such, the EMS provider would not typically be eligible to receive payments by insurance plans unless a patient is transported. This effectively kept the profession in a box, until now.

EMS providers have not only the opportunity, but the responsibility as well, to expand their roles as providers of healthcare to more than emergency transportation. As part of a coordinated effort with doctors and hospitals, EMS providers will be able to respond to patients with a broader range of medical needs in their community. The profession can now be proactive in the approach to mobile integrated healthcare rather than reactive using the traditional 9-1-1 response methods used today throughout the industry. The finance reform of healthcare opens new doors of opportunity for EMS.

Accountable Care Organizations

One of the most talked about provisions of the ACA is the framework under which accountable care organizations (ACO) are created. Simply stated, an ACO is a group of doctors, hospitals, and other healthcare providers who come together voluntarily to give coordinated high-quality care to Medicare patients. The goal of coordinated care is to ensure that patients, especially the chronically ill, receive the right care at the right time, while avoiding unnecessary duplication of services and preventing medical errors.

When an ACO succeeds both in both delivering high-quality care and spending healthcare dollars more wisely, the organization will share in the savings it achieves for the Medicare program.[2] This means that providers who have not been eligible to receive payments from insurance plans now have the opportunity to implement healthcare delivery changes that meet the IHI Triple Aim® and, if so, share in the cost savings.

Integrated Delivery Systems

The same economic incentive model is true for new integrated delivery systems (IDS). For example, Highmark Blue Cross & Blue Shield recently purchased the Allegheny Health System in western Pennsylvania. Why would the largest payer also want to become the largest provider of healthcare services in western Pennsylvania? The answer is control. They will be able to not only manage the patient population, but also manage the costs of delivering care to that population. This system has dramatically changed the healthcare landscape in western Pennsylvania.

ACO and IDS Implications for EMS

The typical payers for EMS are changing. Accountable care in some form is here to stay, and it's rapidly changing the financing of healthcare services. For example, accountable care organizations are given financial incentives to improve patient care and reduce costs. Typically, these goals are achieved by navigating the right patient, to the right resource, at the right time, at the right outcome, at the right cost. In some cases, this involves avoiding the use of a high-cost ambulance to transport the patient to the emergency department as has been traditionally done in the past. An EMS coordinator at the hospital engaged in an ACO will no longer be asking why they are not receiving more patients, but instead may be asking why they are receiving so many patients.

Bundled Payments for Care Improvement Initiative

Traditionally, Medicare makes separate payments to providers for each service they provide to beneficiaries for a single illness or course of treatment. This approach can result in fragmented care with minimal coordination across providers and health care settings. This type of payment scheme rewards the quantity and not the quality of services offered by providers.

There are four bundled payment models:

- In Model 1, the episode of care is defined as the inpatient stay in the acute care hospital. Medicare will pay the hospital a discounted amount based on the payment rates established under the Inpatient Prospective Payment System used in the original Medicare program. Medicare will continue to pay physicians separately for their services under the Medicare Physician Fee Schedule. Under certain circumstances, hospitals and physicians will be permitted to share gains arising from the providers' care redesign efforts.

- In Model 2, the episode of care will include the inpatient stay in the acute care hospital and all related services during the episode. The episode will end either 30, 60, or 90 days after hospital discharge. Participants can select up to 48 different clinical condition episodes.

- In Model 3, the episode of care will be triggered by an acute care hospital stay and will begin at initiation of postacute care services with a participating skilled nursing facility, inpatient rehabilitation facility, long-term care hospital, or home health agency. The postacute care services included in the episode must begin within 30 days of discharge from the inpatient stay and will end either a minimum of 30, 60, or 90 days after the initiation of the episode.

- In Model 4, the Centers for Medicare and Medicaid Services (CMS) will make a single, prospectively determined bundled payment to the hospital that would encompass all services furnished during the inpatient stay by the hospital, physicians, and other practitioners. Physicians and other practitioners will submit "no-pay" claims to Medicare and will be paid by the hospital out of the bundled payment. Related readmissions for 30 days after hospital discharge will be included in the bundled payment amount.

In January 2013 Medicare announced 450 hospitals had been approved to test a new bundled payment program under the Bundled Payments for Care Improvement (BPCI) initiative.[3] The news release provided by the CMS included the following quote:

> *Under the Bundled Payments for Care Improvement initiative, organizations will enter into payment arrangements that include financial and performance accountability for episodes of care. These models may lead to higher-quality, more coordinated care at a lower cost to Medicare.*

It is possible that the IHI Triple Aim initiative is one of the main reasons that Medicare is promoting the bundled payment program. Here's why. Take the example of a patient who falls and suffers a fractured hip. The receiving hospital receives a single payment for the episode of care and is now responsible for paying for all the care relating to that admission, x-rays, labs, surgery, prescriptions, room costs, everything. The hospital is now incentivized to meet the Triple Aim in the following ways:

- Improve the patient experience of care (including quality and satisfaction):
  - The hospital will focus on improving the quality of care (no medical errors and no healthcare-acquired conditions that may lengthen the patient's stay) to reduce the length of stay and associated unnecessary costs.
  - The hospital will also ensure the healing process is accelerated by providing the patient the emotional support and rest necessary. This treatment leads to an enhanced experience of care.

- Improve the health of populations:
  - The hospital is also now motivated to ensure the patient is cared for properly after discharge to prevent an unnecessary readmission for the same episode of care. The hospital may coordinate the transition of the patient to a home or skilled nursing rehabilitation facility to minimize postdischarge infections, falls, or even bed sores that may necessitate a readmission. The care the patient receives outside of the hospital is designed to prevent readmissions, improving the health of populations.

■ Reduce per capita cost:

- When the cost of inpatient and postacute care is less due to the focus on meeting the Triple Aim initiative, the result is a lower cost of care.

In Model 2, one of the most prevalent bundled payment models, the episode of care will include the inpatient stay in an acute-care hospital and all related services during the episode. The episode will end either 30, 60, or 90 days after hospital discharge.

Bundled Payment Implications for EMS

Imagine that the payer for EMS 30, 60, or 90 days after hospital discharge is the hospital that has received the total bundled payment for the patient's course of care. The EMS system may now need to prove to the *hospital* that there is value in the services EMS personnel provided in order to receive payment. How will providers do that? Perhaps by administering the appropriate patient care that prevented the need for a high-cost transport by ambulance to the emergency department. Research has shown that bundled payments can align incentives for providers—hospitals, postacute care providers, doctors, and other practitioners—allowing them to work closely together across all specialties and settings.

Satisfaction-Based Reimbursement

Another significant change in this new healthcare environment is the focus on the patient's experience of care through satisfaction-based reimbursement. Under the ACA and resulting CMS rules, 30% of a hospital's bonus payments are based on patient satisfaction, or the patient's experience of care. This focus has led to the rise of a new *C* suite position, referred to often as the chief experience officer, or the CXO. In hospitals, the person in this position is responsible for maximizing patient satisfaction. CXOs are typically coming from organizations that are experts in customer service and hospitality, such as the hotel industry.

A transformation in leadership has been brought about by the new approach to healthcare.

The Cleveland Clinic was the first major academic medical center to establish an Office of Patient Experience, focused on maximizing patient satisfaction. The Baylor, Scott, & White health system in Fort Worth shared recently that a person has been hired in the marketing department to focus on monitoring the Internet, Twitter, and Facebook to promote awareness of positive comments as well as any negative comments that need to be addressed.

On July 20, 2013, the *Los Angeles Times*[4] detailed the efforts undertaken by San Francisco General Hospital with regard to improving the patient's experience of care:

> Now, patients at San Francisco General Hospital are greeted by a smiling face and a helping hand to guide them along the path to getting care. It's one of a series of customer-friendly touches being added at the 156-year-old institution by a newly named "chief patient experience officer."

"The first questions patients are asked shouldn't be whether they are insured and have an advance directive for end-of-life treatment," said Duffy, who works with San Francisco General and dozens of other hospitals.

"It just takes one person to destroy great outcomes," she said. "It's often the apathetic, rude person at check-in." To help make patients feel more welcome, San Francisco General created the position of director of first impressions.

Satisfaction-Based Payment Implications for EMS

The EMS system can have an impact on a hospital's patient satisfaction scores. If a patient response to the care given by an EMS provider is positive, it may favorably affect the patient satisfaction survey score given to the discharging hospital. Similarly, if a patient does not have a positive experience with the care received from an EMS provider, the patient may link the experience to the discharging hospital and give the hospital a poor rating. This rating may have a financial impact on the hospital because 30% of the VBP bonus or penalty is connected to patient satisfaction. In the new patient-centered healthcare environment with integrated services, providing an excellent customer experience is crucial. The EMS system partnership with hospitals will require reassurance to the hospital that the care by EMS personnel will not only provide a positive outcome but reduce the overall costs to the system.

Managed Medicare and Medicaid Programs

The national push to enroll Medicaid patients into managed care took center stage in Florida in 2013. For years the Florida Agency for Health Care Administration has tried to enroll Medicaid recipients into managed Medicaid programs. That effort was fought by the providers and patients.

Florida wanted to be able to move these patients into managed Medicaid programs because of a significant improvement in the quality of care and a reduction in costs. In June 2013 the federal government gave final approval for this long-debated proposal to move all of the Florida Medicaid patients into managed care plans.[5]

The same situation is happening with Medicare beneficiaries. Part of the managed care movement is to change Medicare from a fee-for-service (FFS) payer to a managed care program. ACOs are already becoming pervasive and may be an interim step on the way to a more efficient American healthcare system.

Chas Roades, chief research officer at the Advisory Board Company in Washington, DC, explained in a recent interview[6] with *Kaiser Health News* that "ACOs aren't the end game." One of the key challenges for hospitals and doctors is that the incentives are to reduce hospital stays, emergency department visits, and expensive specialist and testing services—all the ways that hospitals and doctors make money in the current fee-for-service system. Ultimately, Roades says the goal would be for providers to take on full financial responsibility for caring for a population of patients for a fixed payment, but that will require a transition beyond an ACO. The comment "taking full financial responsibility" sounds a lot like managed care.

VOICES OF EXPERIENCE

It has been awesome to me. Grateful that y'all have been here to talk to and teach me about my medical condition. It's been a blessing that y'all have been here. I never knew this program existed. Y'all have been there to keep me out of the hospital by helping me utilize the healthcare system outside the ER and the hospital. Y'all have been a big help getting me into appointments that I need, and I don't think I could have done myself. I feel that I will be able to do better managing my own healthcare with the information and teachings that y'all have provided.

Laketha Allen
MedStar MIH patient

Managed Medicare and Medicaid Program Implications for EMS

EMS providers who are accustomed to billing the state for Medicaid patients are now more often billing a managed care payer for Medicare or Medicaid patients. It could well be that in the near future, EMS will be paid by a small number of managed care companies who are fully financially responsible for Medicare, Medicaid, and commercial plan patients. The managed care payers may have a much different set of value measures than a state agency.

CMS Bonuses and Penalties for Hospitals

Currently, CMS provides financial bonuses or penalties to hospitals based on value-based purchasing and readmission rates. From a government perspective and from a budgetary perspective, this program is attractive because it changes behavior through financial incentives and is budget neutral.

Value-based purchasing is a payment methodology based on quality metrics such as clinical outcomes, patient satisfaction, and other quality standards. Metrics monitor the adherence to the standards. A system of rewards and consequences is applied, conditional upon prespecified performance standards. If hospitals demonstrate excellence on key measures, they receive bonuses on their Medicare reimbursement. If hospitals fall below established standards, their payments are reduced. **Table 2-1** shows some of the clinical quality performance metrics on which hospitals are being evaluated.

Table 2-1 Measures of Clinical Quality Performance

Clinical Process of Care Measures	
Measure ID	**Measure Description**
Acute Myocardial Infarction (AMI)	
AMI-7a	Fibrinolytic Therapy Received Within 30 Minutes of Hospital Arrival
AMI-8a	Primary Percutaneous Coronary Intervention (PCI) Received Within 90 Minutes of Hospital Arrival
Heart Failure (HF)	
HF-1	Discharge Instructions
Survey Measures	
Measure ID	**Measure Description**
HCAHPS	Hospital Consumer Assessment of Healthcare Providers and Systems Survey

Reproduced from: Centers for Medicare & Medicaid Services. Hospital value-based purchasing.

Note the measure AMI-8a. EMS providers have encouraged the investment in technology to enable them to send 12-lead ECGs and call STEMI alerts from the field to the hospital. Current research reveals that clinically, time matters for patients experiencing an ST-elevation myocardial infarction.[7] CMS is therefore using the 90-minute door to balloon time as a measure of clinical excellence. If the hospital fails to meet these clinical goals, significant amounts of revenue are at risk.

Consequently, hospitals are working on collaborative solutions, including purchasing 12-lead transfer stations or other similar devices, to ensure compliance with clinical metrics. **Table 2-2** depicts the domains and weights of penalties or bonuses, and **Table 2-3** shows a sample of survey scores.

Table 2-2 Scoring of Penalties or Bonuses

FY 2014 Scoring	
Domain	**Weight**
Clinical Process of Care	45%
Patient Experience of Care	30%
Outcome Mortality	25%
FY 2015 Scoring	
Domain	**Weight**
Clinical Process of Care	20%
Patient Experience of Care	30%
Outcome	30%
Efficiency	20%

Data from: Hospital value-based purchasing scoring/QualityNet.

Table 2-3 Sample Survey Scores for Select Providers, 2014

Provider Number	Communication with Nurses Achievement Points	Responsiveness of Hospital Staff Achievement Points	Pain Management Achievement Points	HCAHPS Base Score
010001	3 out of 10	0 out of 10	3 out of 10	35
010005	8 out of 10	3 out of 10	7 out of 10	53
010006	2 out of 10	0 out of 10	0 out of 10	8
010011	2 out of 10	2 out of 10	1 out of 10	14
010012	3 out of 10	5 out of 10	5 out of 10	25
010019	4 out of 10	4 out of 10	3 out of 10	37
010021	5 out of 10	0 out of 10	5 out of 10	28
010023	3 out of 10	4 out of 10	1 out of 10	25
010024	5 out of 10	3 out of 10	5 out of 10	43
010025	4 out of 10	6 out of 10	0 out of 10	25
010029	5 out of 10	5 out of 10	4 out of 10	53
010033	6 out of 10	3 out of 10	4 out of 10	42

Note: HCAHPS, Hospital Consumer Assessment of Healthcare Providers and Systems.
Data from: HCAHPS.

CMS also provides financial bonuses or penalties to hospitals based on 30-day readmission rates for select diagnosis-related groups (DRGs), such as congestive heart failure (CHF) and myocardial infarction (**Table 2-4**). CMS has focused on CHF because it represents the largest expense for Medicare—14% of Medicare beneficiaries have a diagnosis of CHF, but it represents 43% of all Medicare expenditures.[8]

Table 2-4 Sample Readmission Penalties for Select Providers

FY 2014 IPPS Final Rule: Hospital Readmissions Reduction Program-Supplemental Data							
PROV	FY 2014 Readmissions Adjustment Factor	Number of Pneumonia Cases	Excess Readmission Ratio for Pneumonia	Number of Heart Failure Cases	Excess Readmission Ratio for Heart Failure	Number of Acute Myocardial Infarction Cases	Acute Myocardial Infarction Excess Readmission Ratio
010001	1.0000	368	0.968954	901	0.912972	747	0.980807
010005	1.0000	331	0.937659	248	0.945339	18	0.000000
010006	1.0000	793	0.942541	652	0.824785	310	0.927480
010007	0.9944	220	1.043892	115	1.068507	5	0.000000
010008	1.0000	57	0.981442	51	0.989199	4	0.000000
010009	0.9981	88	1.025793	109	1.007290	9	0.000000
010010	0.9972	291	1.054462	150	0.950906	10	0.000000
010011	0.9999	484	0.973534	388	0.903865	239	1.002744
010012	0.9969	240	0.955323	148	1.076317	85	1.035684
010016	0.9981	331	0.934693	309	1.020497	234	1.040508
010018	1.0000	0	0.000000	0	0.000000	0	0.000000

Note: Values less than 1 represent penalties. Values greater than 1 represent bonuses.
Data from: Centers for Disease Control and Prevention.

One hospital admission for CHF costs Medicare an average of $21,489,[9] with a national 30-day readmission rate of 24.7%, and 52% of the patients who are readmitted within 30 days did not see their primary care physician between discharge and readmission. The Medicare Payment Advisory Commission (MedPAC) estimates that $12 billion per year is spent on potentially preventable readmissions.[10]

For fiscal year 2013–2014 (October–September), the maximum potential value-based purchasing and readmission penalties for hospitals is 3%, which is applied to every Medicare admission. For example, if a hospital generates $100 million in Medicare fees and is assessed a 1.5% penalty on every Medicare dollar, their annual penalty is $1.5 million. Most hospitals operate on a 2–3% profit margin at best. Reductions in payments therefore have the potential to change a hospital from being marginally profitable to maybe breaking even or operating in the red (**Table 2-5**).

Table 2-5 Value-Based Purchasing and Readmission Penalties for Select Hospitals in Tennessee

Hospital	City	VBP%	Admit%	Total%
Vanderbilt University Hospital	Nashville	−0.15%	−0.60%	−0.75%
Methodist Healthcare Memphis	Memphis	0.13%	−0.78%	−0.65%
Cumberland Medical Center	Crossville	−0.43%	−1.00%	−1.43%
Johnson City Medical Center	Johnson City	−0.08%	−1.00%	−1.08%

Data from: MedPAC. Payment policy for inpatient readmissions. Report to Congress: promoting greater efficiency in medicare. June 2001.

An article in the December 2012 edition of *Modern Healthcare* illustrates this point from the perspective a hospital executive.[11]

In 2013, Henry Ford Health System projects to lose $2.2 million from readmissions with $1 million of those losses coming from Henry Ford Hospital.

Those cuts for the Henry Ford system will increase in 2014 to $4.3 million, including $2 million at Henry Ford Hospital, because the penalties will increase to 2% in 2014 and 3% in 2015.

Despite reducing actual readmission rates, Detroit Medical Center expects to lose $1.7 million, or 0.8% of Medicare payments, by not meeting the strict readmission standards, said Dee Prosi, DMC's senior vice president of marketing and business development.

Dearborn-based Oakwood Hospital and Medical Center stands to lose $1.2 million in 2013, or 0.82% of base Medicare reimbursement, according to an Oakwood statement.

St. John Providence Health System expects to lose $2.3 million in fiscal 2013, despite making progress in reducing readmissions, CFO Pat McGuire said.

Healthcare finance reform has become a significant financial problem for hospitals. Hospitals need to develop programs and partnerships with doctors and EMS providers to coordinate and integrate services to improve the healthcare system and turn penalties into bonuses.

For example, an April 2013 article in the *New York Times*[12] chronicled a new way physicians are working with hospitals to reduce potentially preventable readmissions:

> *Chicago—On a stormy evening this spring, nurses at Dr. Gary Stuck's family practice were on the phone with patients with heart ailments, asking them not to shovel snow. The idea was to keep them out of the hospital, and that effort—combined with dozens more like it—is starting to make a difference: across the city, doctors are providing less, but not worse, health care.... Under the agreement, hospital admissions are down 6%. Days spent in the hospital are down nearly 9%.*
>
> *The average length of a stay has declined, and many other measures show doctors providing less care, too.*

Dr. Stuck is most likely given a financial incentive to reduce hospital readmissions, which is why he is willing to have his staff call patients advising them not to shovel snow and risk a possible heart attack. Healthcare is changing.

Bonus and Penalty Implications for EMS

If a hospital is concerned about its readmission rates for CHF, myocardial infarction, or other conditions, it may be receptive to partnering with EMS on a program that safely reduces potentially preventable readmissions. At MedStar, a successful CHF program is currently being funded by one of the local hospitals. With the implementation of the ACA, additional incentives have been created that make mobile integrated healthcare programs much more attractive.

In addition to connecting frequent users of the emergency department with appropriate resources for their healthcare needs, improving the patient's experience with the healthcare system, and lowering costs, the programs stand to transform healthcare processes and encourage collaboration. Where there is current fragmentation, mobile integrated healthcare programs facilitate connections and improving communication between healthcare providers, patients, and the communities in which they live.

Federal and Legislative Initiatives Supporting MIH

In their 2006 *EMS at the Crossroads*, the Institute of Medicine (IOM) identified critical challenges facing field EMS. These challenges included insufficient coordination, disparities in response times, and a lack of readiness and inadequate federal funding for disaster preparedness.[13] Improving the quality of care and innovation and strengthening field EMS at the state, federal, and local levels is now the focus. The Field EMS Quality, Innovation, Cost-Effectiveness Improvement Act (H.R. 809), introduced by Rep. Larry Bucshon (R-IN), addresses these challenges affecting EMS. The legislation would address the systemic problems plaguing EMS by implementing key IOM recommendations—including the designation of the Department of Health and Human Services (HHS) as the primary federal agency for the integration of EMS within the larger health system. This appointment would ensure continuity of care from the patient's perspective. The bill would also enhance federal support for EMS agencies, states, and educational entities, and for EMS research to promote high-quality field EMS. The new legislation does not add to the federal deficit because new programs would be funded by voluntary contributions made by taxpayers when filing their federal income tax forms. As the industry tests new EMS delivery methods and payment models, they will be centered on improving outcomes and lowering costs.

Finance Reform and the World of EMS

When Medicare ties its reimbursement rates to VPB measures, EMS providers will have to adjust how they do business as an industry to survive financially. The new model requires innovative thought and leadership transformation. EMS, both public and private services, will not survive with the old mantra of "You call. We haul." EMS organizations and leaders will have to be prepared to make a shift by asking themselves whether they are ready to transform their business processes in order to create a service-based, patient-centered healthcare organization. Those that do can not only survive, but thrive!

American healthcare and EMS system executives and leadership need to embrace delivery system transformation. Charles Kennedy, the CEO of ACS, Accountable Care Solutions, said in an article in *Hospitals and Health Network* magazine, "We are selecting partners with executive leadership that sees the same type of change that we think is possible. Much like venture capitalists, we are investing in the leadership team.[14]" Leaders in EMS must ask themselves, "Am I that type of transformational leader?"

Pearls of WISDOM

H.R. 809, The Field EMS Quality, Innovation, and Cost Effectiveness Improvements Act of 2013, better known as the Field EMS Bill, allows numerous enhancements to occur for EMS and MIH programs. Among other things, it designates the lead federal agency for EMS in the Department of Health and Human Services, the same department as CMS and the Assistant Secretary for Preparedness and Response. The Field EMS Bill also facilitates the testing of alternate economic models for EMS. Read and become familiar with this bill. If you agree with the initiatives, Join the National Association of EMTs and numerous legislative sponsors to pass the bill in Congress. The bill is available at: http://beta.congress.gov/bill/113th-congress/house-bill/809.

Are You READY?

- Read the IOM *EMS at the Crossroads* report from 2006 at: http://www.iom.edu/Reports/2006/Emergency-Medical-Services-At-the-Crossroads.aspx.

- Read the EMS Agenda for the Future from 1996 at: http://www.ems.gov/pdf/2010/EMSAgendaWeb_7-06-10.pdf.

- Research the Institute for Healthcare Improvement Triple Aim initiative at: http://www.ihi.org/Engage/Initiatives/TripleAim/Pages/default.aspx.

Summary

Mobile resources that are integrated with the healthcare system can positively and dramatically impact the patient's outcome, their experience of care, and reduce costs, thereby meeting the IHI Triple Aim. Mobile integrated healthcare programs reduce unnecessary hospital use through patient education and communication and improve chronically ill patient care and hospice services. The patient experience is improved as a result.

Currently, our healthcare system is bankrupting the country. Positive changes are welcome and will help increase public satisfaction and expectation about high-quality healthcare. A solid foundation is the beginning. It is also important to understand how the opportunities created by the healthcare finance reforms brought about by the ACA create opportunities for EMS to operate and provide quality out-of-hospital care in a whole new way within the healthcare system.

References

1. Institute for Healthcare Improvement. Initiatives: The IHI Triple Aim. Available at: http://www .ihi.org/Engage/Initiatives/TripleAim/Pages/default.aspx. Accessed May 12, 2014.

2. Centers for Medicare & Medicaid Services. Shared savings program. Available at: http://www .cms.gov/Medicare/Medicare-Fee-for-Service-Payment/ACO/index.html?redirect=/aco/. Accessed May 12, 2014.

3. Centers for Medicare & Medicaid Services. Fact sheets: Bundled payments for care improvement initiative. Available at: FR http://www.cms.gov/Newsroom/MediaReleaseDatabase/ Fact-Sheets/2014-Fact-sheets-items/2014-01-30-2.html. Accessed May 12, 2014.

4. Gorman A. Healthcare overhaul leads hospitals to focus on patient satisfaction. *Los Angeles Times*. July 20, 2013. Available at: http://articles.latimes.com/2013/jul/20/local/la-me-patient-satisfaction-20130721. Accessed May 12, 2014.

5. Saunders J. Capsules: The KHN blog. Florida's win: Feds grant Medicaid managed care waiver. *Kaiser Health News*. June 14, 2013. Available at: http://capsules.kaiserhealthnews.org/index .php/2013/06/floridas-victory-feds-grant-medicaid-managed-care-waiver/. Accessed May 12, 2014.

6. Gold J. FAQ on ACOs: Accountable care organizations, explained. *Kaiser Health News*. April 16, 2014. Available at: http://www.kaiserhealthnews.org/stories/2011/january/13/aco-accountable-care-organization-faq.aspx. Accessed May 12, 2014.

7. O'Gara PT, Kushner FG, Ascheim DD, et al. ACCF/AHA guideline for the management of ST-elevation myocardial infarction: Executive summary: A report of the American College of Cardiology Foundation/American Heart Association Task Force on Practice Guidelines; *Circ J*. December 2012.

8. Centers for Medicaid & Medicare Services. Medicare. Available at: http://www.cms.gov/ Medicare/Medicare-General-Information/CCIP/index.html?redirect=/CCIP/. Accessed May 12, 2014.

9. Centers for Disease Control and Prevention. Heart failure fact sheet. Available at: http:// www.cdc.gov/dhdsp/data_statistics/fact_sheets/docs/fs_heart_failure.pdf. Accessed May 12, 2014.

10. MedPAC. Payment policy for inpatient readmissions. Report to Congress: Promoting greater efficiency in Medicare. June 2001. Available at: http://www.medpac.gov/chapters/jun07_ch05 .pdf. Accessed May 12, 2014.

11. Greene J. Hospitals face reimbursement penalties over readmission rates. *Modern Healthcare*. Available at: http://www.modernhealthcare.com/article/20121210/INFO/312109979. Accessed May 12, 2014.

12. Lowrey A. A health provider strives to keep hospital beds empty. *The New York Times*. April 23, 2013. Available at: http://www.nytimes.com/2013/04/24/business/accountable-care-helping-hospitals-keep-medical-costs-down.html?_r=0. Accessed May 12, 2014.

13. Institute of Medicine. Emergency medical services at the crossroads. June 13, 2006. Available at: http://www.iom.edu/Reports/2006/Emergency-Medical-Services-At-the-Crossroads.aspx. Accessed May 12, 2014.

14. Weinstock M. Don't be a wallflower: Hospital executives must become agents of change or miss out on the opportunities that lie ahead. *Hospitals and Health Networks*. August 1, 2013. Available at: http://www.hhnmag.com/display/HHN-news-article.dhtml?dcrPath=/templatedata/HF_Common/NewsArticle/data/HHN/Magazine/2013/Aug/0813HHN_healthmatters. Accessed May 12, 2014.

3

Organizational Readiness Assessment

A model mobile integrated healthcare (MIH) program is developed based upon a series of internal and external assessments.

How to Begin

The first two chapters outlined the healthcare landscape and the benefits for EMS to transition to a quality, patient-centered mobile integrated healthcare model. By now you're motivated to learn how the transformation can be made from an EMS system into a mobile integrated healthcare program. Your entire organization needs to embrace the change. First, determine whether or not *your organization* is ready to make this transformation. It doesn't matter whether your organization is large or small, private or public, fire based or hospital based—it all starts at the first step of determining whether the leadership of the organization is averse to risk or willing to be transformational.

A risk-averse organization is one that is satisfied with the status quo, happy living in the moment in a safe, secure environment it knows and can understand. History is replete with examples of organizations that were unable to take risks to transform, and as such, now face difficult times, or at least missed opportunities:

- Blockbuster—Once an iconic video superstore, it missed the opportunity to move into the mail order and video-on-demand distribution opportunities.

- Eastman/Kodak—Once on the verge of complete domination of the photo industry, it failed to transition to the digital platform.

- Yahoo—It had the opportunity to become the premier Internet search engine, only to be eclipsed by Google.

If your organization is averse to risk, you may have to educate others and perhaps even lobby others, such as your senior leadership or executive team, to help gain support for mobile integrated healthcare. If you're in a position to lead this process for your organization, then knowing potential objections that may be raised by your leadership team is crucial. Some of the more common objections are the lack of demonstrated sustainable revenue, the counterintuitive concept of implementing programs to actually reduce transport volume, and the ever-present "That's not the way we have always done it."

The journey is long and complex, but this text provides some of the best strategies for a successful transition and the specific steps MedStar has taken to create an MIH program. You and your team need to become students of healthcare during one of the most dynamic times not only in the EMS profession, but in the entire healthcare system. Be aware of the changes that have already occurred and those likely to happen in the future. Spend time educating yourself on the most recent healthcare initiatives, and read healthcare periodicals to be informed. Knowledge of the current state of health care and EMS will help you prepare for change and to communicate effectively with healthcare partners. This expertise will be crucial in the decades to come and will help your organization change the way it needs to in order to meet this new healthcare opportunity. You may have an innovative workforce and progressive leadership, or you may have a very traditional organization and leadership that tends to be resistant to change. Regardless of the type of culture you have, the future of your organization and the future of your community and the way emergency medical services are delivered to your community are changing. Successful EMS providers will be able to quickly adapt. The success of the program hinges on internal and external communication and willingness to participate.

All stakeholders must actively believe and buy into the concept of the MIH program and the need for it. Once you've received buy-in internally, begin dialogue with the external stakeholders.

Internal Stakeholders

Medical Directors

In the new healthcare environment, there is a significant clinical component, and strong support from EMS medical directors will be crucial. At MedStar, a progressive medical director, Steven Davis, MD, EMT-P, is committed to innovative approaches to healthcare and is driving many of the changes. Dr. Davis promotes the MedStar mobile healthcare program to his professional constituents, and several of the MIH programs being done at MedStar are the direct result of Dr. Davis's initiatives.

Conversations with your medical director will help assess whether or not your organization is ready to head down this new path. You may also find it beneficial to suggest that the medical director speak with others who have been involved in establishing MIH programs. There are number of physician leaders in this movement who can speak doctor to doctor with your medical director to provide input and guidance. Some of the physician leaders of the MIH movement are:

Brent Myers, MD, MPH, FACEP; Wake County, North Carolina

Michael Wilcox, MD; Hopkins, Minnesota

Ed Racht, MD; American Medical Response/Envision Healthcare

Eric Beck, DO, NREMT-P; American Medical Response/Envision Healthcare

James Dunford, MD; San Diego, California

Gary Smith, MD; Mesa, Arizona

Determine whether the physician medical director is committed to developing, implementing, coordinating, and evaluating the MIH program. Examples of active participation include helping to understand community healthcare needs; writing protocols, policies, and procedures; and participating in the facilitation of meetings to foster stakeholder engagement. The medical director needs to be involved in all aspects of the program, including training, provider selection, quality assurance, and the evaluation of program goals and objectives.

Senior Leadership

The next step in the internal assessment of organizational readiness to provide mobile integrated healthcare is to talk with your senior leadership team. It's important that any governing board members, advisory board members, and executive team members understand how this type of program will benefit the organization, its patients, and the community.

To thrive in this new environment, you will need to talk to your workforce and explain why mobile integrated healthcare is important. Start with the labor union leadership, if applicable, and get internal buy-in as you did with your board of directors, your executive director, medical director, and others throughout the entire organization. When internal stakeholders understand the benefits of an MIH program, they'll support the process. EMS providers will have a larger role in patient care and presence in the community, helping alleviate some of the staff workloads, and increase the revenue of their organization.

First Responders

First responders are a very important link in the MIH delivery process. In many communities, first responders are first to receive the call for help as the primary public safety answering point (PSAP) and/or the patient's first contact with the EMS system.

In Fort Worth, Texas, the role of first responders is evolving in this new delivery system model. For example, in the MedStar 9-1-1 nurse triage program, there would be times that the first responders arrived on scene when the nurse was still on the phone with the caller.

Typically, once MedStar providers arrive on scene, they are able to relieve the first responders if the patient's condition is stable. This response is documented as "relieved by MedStar on scene," and the first responders are not required to obtain patient release signatures. This is a crucial part of MedStar's system to help ensure that first responders are available to provide a rapid response to other emergency calls. The medical director enabled the emergency medical responders to clear the scene by allowing them to use the same process if MedStar's triage nurse is on the phone with the caller assisting with an alternate disposition for the patient, which in most cases is being done without a response from an ambulance.

First-response organizations are under pressure to become more economically efficient and generate revenue in new ways. First responders such as EMT/fire fighters may be an integral part of your mobile integrated healthcare program. MIH providers, however, can be from all levels of certification or licensure. Patient wellness checks can be performed by emergency medical responders or EMTs. An EMT, for example, could check on a diabetic patient in-between emergency calls or during a regular shift to remind the patient to check her blood sugar level (or even check it for her if permitted in your state or region) or to make sure that she has eaten. Patient wellness and care within the home is all part of MIH.

External Stakeholders

Once the internal agency assessment, or system organizational readiness assessment, is done, the external stakeholders need to be addressed. You need to determine how your organization is perceived in the community.

Hospital Partners and Other Healthcare Organizations

Evaluate your relationship with your hospital partners and other medical leaders in the community. To be successful, an MIH program will need to integrate with hospitals, local or county physician medical societies, skilled nursing facilities, home health agencies, hospice agencies, primary care practices, and clinics.

Conduct an environmental assessment to determine the external issues facing the healthcare organizations in your community, especially with regard to value-based purchasing bonuses or penalties, readmission bonuses or penalties, and other healthcare industry changes that have an effect on them.

EMS providers can bridge the gap and provide solutions, but it is important to build allies first. In Fort Worth, relationships with the entire healthcare community were developed through MedStar's medical control board, the emergency physicians advisory board, and through many of the hospital leaders in the community. MedStar personnel accomplished this by working on joint projects and public health initiatives, serving on task forces, and regularly scheduling briefing meetings with members of the local healthcare community.

As with anything else, you need relationships to prosper and grow. Lay the groundwork, and prepare for the right conversations at the right time. If you've already built a strong foundation of trust with stakeholders it becomes easier to bring the concept of MIH to them. If you don't have those relationships, start building that trust now!

Organizational Inclusivity

When MedStar began to think about treating their EMS loyalty program members (patients who use 9-1-1 15 or more times in 90 days) in a different way, a summit was convened at the facility and many external stakeholders were invited. The initial meeting invitations included everyone

At Kaiser Permanente Northwest, I see expansion of our delivery system in the area of prehospital care, integral to and aligned with our mission to transform care and achieve the Triple Aim goals. In Kaiser's experience, four key points have been found to be critical to exploring and ultimately integrating the EMS system into the hospital delivery system.

First, Kaiser's system and ambulance partners had medical directors who were open to innovation and had the courage to explore possibilities. Having an understanding of the scope and skills of the EMTs, Kaiser's team was able to develop and share with senior leaders what and where the value of EMS could be for Kaiser Permanente. In addition, Kaiser's vision was in alignment with the ambulance medical director, which helped serve as the foundation for trust between our two complex systems. Having a key point person, with a highly accountable team in Kaiser Permanente, helped shepherd communication, build trust, and develop a deep understanding of the value for the Northwest care delivery teams.

Second, Kaiser recognized that there is a tremendous information gap between hospital- and clinic-based care teams, and the scope and skills of the EMS and prehospital care teams. In order to close that gap and build trust, the Plan, Do, See, Act methodology was used. By using a series of PDSAs, a much greater understanding, respect, and team strength was developed to launch our expansion and to see past the traditional "Johnny and Roy" perception of EMS providers.

Third, EMS systems are very complex, full of regulations, politics, and misdirected incentives that, on first glance, would intimidate the most determined director. By looking for small possibilities and taking small steps that centered on the needs of the patient and health care system, pathways to success became clear, making alignment easier, and increasing the chances for others to see successful opportunities and value.

Last, adopt the philosophy of not reinventing the wheel and partnering with organizations that have a successful model. EMS systems may be different, but the clinical practice of medicine remains the same regardless of the community. Sharing and implementing existing best practices, making modifications to fit your system's needs or resources will save you time, energy, and money, and will increase your chance for success. Working with the team at MedStar, continuing to learn from each other, and sharing experiences, has accelerated our organization's learning in this developing area. Kaiser's partnership with organizations like MedStar, who are willing to share their programs, and what they learned along the way, has helped us avoid common pitfalls and improved our implementation strategy.

Rahul Rostogi, MD
*Director of Operations for Continuing Care
    Services and Quality Value Management*
Kaiser Permanente
*Northwest Permanente, PC, Physicians &
    Surgeons*
Portland, OR

from hospital representatives, to large physician practices, to representatives from the nursing organizations, first response agencies, home health agencies, clinic providers, the Area Agency on Aging, the United Way, and the local mental health organizations. The invitations shared the list of invitees, who were asked to extend invitations to any other agency or stakeholder group not on the list they believed might also want to be part of the initial discussions.

At this breakfast meeting, dialogue began about caring for the EMS loyalty program members in a way that was more patient centered and used healthcare resources in a more coordinated manner to improve patient health. MedStar providers wanted to reach out and conduct home visits and try to connect these patients with resources in the community, and external stakeholders were invited to share their ideas on what some of those connections might look like. Key constituency groups were willing to share their counsel because MedStar personnel had invested time over the years building those relationships. They trusted MedStar's decision-making abilities and commitment to solve problems for their agencies and for delivering better care to their patients.

Conducting these types of open discussions is beneficial because all the organizations are hearing the ideas for the first time, together. The collaborative spirit builds when everyone is in the room discussing similar issues. An initial meeting also prevents one hospital or stakeholder group from wondering why they weren't approached first or from feeling left out. It prevents misunderstandings and fosters integration.

Once the initial stakeholder session is done, the groundwork has been laid for individual discussions with the participants. During these meetings, you can determine more specific needs for each stakeholder to determine how you can help meet those needs. MedStar personnel met internally over the course of several weeks to determine how to effectively meet the needs of the stakeholders.

The procedures discussed are part of the assessment of organizational readiness. Were there processes that needed improvement? Were there relationships that needed to be invested in more? What changes needed to be made early to ensure a stronger foundation moving forward? An environmental assessment is a readiness exercise that can strengthen your plan.

MedStar also found that the process energized and strengthened the management team and employee workforce and helped them become excited about getting involved in something new and innovative. There was a buzz going around—employees talking about how to improve patient care, improve outcomes, and potentially reduce the workload on the staff. Once the foundation had been laid and reinforced with the commitment from internal staff and medical directors, MedStar was ready.

Pearls of **WISDOM**

One of the greatest challenges as you head down the MIH route is "mission creep," the inevitable drift into initiating programs that may have a high investment with returns that are difficult to measure. As you assess your organizational readiness, identify a person within your organization who can serve the role of "value police." This key role will continually balance the "can do/should do" scenario, the realist who is far enough removed from the emotional commitment of the programs to be able to help you avoid delving into programs that seem exciting, but might not be a program that you can master to meet the Triple Aim.

Are You **READY?**

- Read the *Readiness Assessment & Developing Project Aims* QI module from the Health Resources and Service Administration at http://www.hrsa.gov/quality/toolbox/methodology/ readinessassessment/.

- Read the book *Strategic Acceleration: Succeed at the Speed of Life*, by Tony Jeary, Vanguard Press, New York, NY, 2009.

- Assemble an "innovation center" at your agency that would include key leaders (executive, operational, clinical) who would evaluate potential innovative ideas based in clinical, operational, and financial efficacy.

Summary

The determination of organizational readiness is an invaluable step in the development of an MIH program. Organizational readiness has to be firmly rooted; otherwise, the weight of the things you learn in the rest of this book will merely serve to crumble the foundation, and the program will collapse.

4

Assessing Community Needs and Promoting Stakeholder Engagement

In Fort Worth, Texas, the implementation of the mobile integrated healthcare program was met with enthusiastic support from the community and the internal and external stakeholders. But that did not happen without the careful foundation of community building as described previously. A successful program takes a lot of hard work, strategic planning, synergistic partnerships, and effective communication.

In the community, MedStar worked with healthcare system stakeholders, city officials, elected officials, case workers, and social service organizations. Partnerships with several nonprofit and for-profit organizations were established. A Care Coordination Council meets monthly to facilitate communication with community-based social service and healthcare organizations to coordinate the clinical and social care that the patients enrolled in the MIH programs need to have to improve outcomes. Continuous communication centered on meeting the needs of current and future patients enrolled in the MIH programs is the best way to foster ongoing relationships with care providers.

MedStar partners in the community include hospitals, physician groups, community service organizations, patients, community leaders, and even elected officials. These partners are aware of the needs that exist, so they support innovation to improve the community's health, and they are wholeheartedly in favor of evolving the traditional EMS system into an MIH program.

Assessing Community Needs

MIH by definition should be integrated into the existing resources available in your community. Any MIH program is only going to be successful if it fills a gap in the resources available in *your* local community. Just because a specific MIH program works in Fort Worth, Texas, or Raleigh-Durham, North Carolina, or Eagle County, Colorado, doesn't mean it will work in your community.

The healthcare needs of urban and rural areas may differ, so it's important to find out from your local community the existing gaps in the provision of healthcare that your program may be able to fill.

This process begins with the community needs assessment, which provides the information necessary for a gap analysis (**Table 4-1**).

Table 4-1 Sample Elements of an MIH Needs Assessment Process

- Identify healthcare issues in the community
  - Hospital readmission rates
  - Inappropriate emergency services use
    - Frequent
    - Low acuity
  - Safety
    - Falls
    - Drowning
  - Pediatric asthma
  - Diabetes
  - Vaccinations
  - Mental health
- Identify prevalent healthcare gaps in access and/or delivery
  - Vulnerable populations and other barriers to healthcare
    - Homeless and mental health patients
    - Children
    - Elderly
    - Mobility barriers
    - Low income and residually uninsured
    - Cultural and language barriers
    - Geographic isolation
  - Influences on the disparities and inequalities in the services offered by the healthcare system
    - Insurance status
    - Languages
    - Lack of provider awareness of a patient's inability to access care
    - Lack of provider awareness of resources
    - Community geographic and socioeconomic factors

Change starts with determining your community's needs. What healthcare services are missing in your area, and what could fill that gap? Who are the right providers to do so, and what knowledge, skills, and abilities do they need? What role could an MIH program serve in bridging gaps in the local community?

Questions You Need to Ask for a Community Needs Assessment

Answer the following questions—this is your *opinion/perception*:

1. What is the one thing about your healthcare system that keeps you up at night? What is your greatest concern?

2. If you had a magic wand and could change one thing, but only one thing about your healthcare system, what would you change (when money and resources are no object)?

3. What are the current barriers to change in your healthcare system?

4. Who is not at the table today who should be (either an agency or person)?

5. What are the top three gaps in your healthcare services?

To assist with finding answers to these questions, the National Association of EMTs convened a Community Paramedicine/MIH committee comprising the following associations:

- The National Association of EMTs

- The American College of Emergency Physicians

- The National Association of EMS Physicians

- The National Association of State EMS Officials

- The National EMS Management Association

- The American Ambulance Association

- The International Academies of Emergency Dispatch

- The International Roundtable on Community Paramedicine

- The North Central EMS Institute

- The Paramedic Foundation

- The National Association of EMS Educators

- The Association of Critical Care Transport

During the collaborative development of a vision statement on MIH and community paramedicine, there was general consensus on the components of a successful mobile integrated healthcare program that have been articulated in a joint vision statement on MIH published by the EMS associations listed above.[1] The 10 pillars to a successful mobile integrated healthcare program, which have been previously described, are as follows:

- Fully integrated

- Collaborative

- Patient centric

- Recognized as the practice of medicine

- Team based

- Educationally appropriate

- Consistent with the IHI Triple Aim philosophy

- Financially sustainable

- Legally compliant

- Supplemental to the existing healthcare system and resources

MedStar agrees that those foundational principles are a good start, and that mobile integrated healthcare can evolve to be even more effective in improving patient care.

Stakeholder Engagement

The evolution of EMS to MIH has fostered one of the most passionate discussions in the profession. In this movement, EMS has the responsibility to engage stakeholders in the evolution and discussion.

Since late 2011, MedStar has hosted site visits for 142 communities in 41 states and 5 foreign nations to share information about MedStar's operations and their MIH services. Additionally, several early MIH adopters from communities such as Wake County, NC; Pittsburg, PA; Eagle County, CO; and northern Minnesota have traveled the country speaking at national, state, and local conferences to help prepare providers and stakeholders for the MIH evolution.

Kaiser Permanente is one of the largest and most innovative integrated healthcare delivery systems in the country. They own 67 hospitals and provide health insurance to 9 million people through their plans. They are a both a *provider of* services and a *payer for* services. Kaiser sent 15 corporate representatives to MedStar for a 2-day education and on-site experience of MIH in action. Kaiser also sent 4 representatives to the 2013 EMS World Mobile Integrated Healthcare Summit.

Why would one of the largest healthcare providers that is also one of the largest payers of services want to learn about MIH? Because, like all providers and payers, they want to improve the healthcare of patients by providing them with the right care, at the right time, in the right setting, with the right outcome at the right cost. Kaiser and MedStar share the same goals. The organizations that EMS should collaborate with share the same frustrations and challenges. Through collaboration, it becomes easier to identify and agree on solutions and approaches to provide higher-quality care and reduce costs.

To gain support and facilitate collaboration, bring together all of your various healthcare and community stakeholders—and don't forget about elected and appointed officials, the media, and any others who may have an interest in this process (**Table 4-2**).

For example, MedStar conducted an initial MIH program that focused on people who were calling 9-1-1 or going to emergency departments for ambulatory care-sensitive (primary care) conditions. This program revealed the importance of communicating with external stakeholders, who not only serve a crucial role in care coordination for patients enrolled in the MIH program, but also who may have been concerned about what MedStar was doing or perceived the MIH program as possibly invading their space in the market. In addition to the obvious desire to identify and collaborate with

VOICES OF EXPERIENCE

Klarus Home Care initiated a collaboration with an EMS agency to help Klarus during nights and weekends and to help them know when one of their enrolled patients calls 9-1-1.

> We are very excited about partnering with MedStar on this program and believe that the high-level emergency resources offered by MedStar will strengthen our ability to more effectively and efficiently respond to patient needs by providing diagnostics and treatment in the home while preventing defaults to care in an emergency room setting, which is significantly more costly and taxing for our patients. The Community Needs Assessment in the Regional Health Care Partnership Plan led by JPS reports that every congestive heart failure (CHF) hospitalization avoided saves the healthcare system some $9,203.00. Patients with CHF frequently visit the emergency room when they become symptomatic and feel short of breath. These are patients who we can easily be evaluated and treated in the home at a fraction of the cost of care delivered in an emergency room setting. It is often as simple as calming a patient's anxieties and providing some needed reassurance.

J. Daniel Bruce, LCSW, CCM, GCM
Administrator
Klarus Home Care

Table 4-2 Recommended Stakeholder List

Stakeholders include individuals, institutions, and organizations that have knowledge about or a potential to have an impact on the health status of the community.

- Medical director(s)
- Hospitals
- Administration
- Case management
- Social work
- Cardiologists
- Home health agencies
- Extended care/skilled nursing facilities
- Hospice agencies
- Internal workforce
- Emergency medical responders
- Healthcare system regulators
- Community-based organizations (e.g., United Way, Meals On Wheels, Catholic Charities, shelters, the Salvation Army)
- Public health agencies
- Clinics (public and private)
- Educational institutions
- Behavioral health agencies
- Health science centers
- Pharmacies
- Third-party payers
- Public officials (elected and appointed)
- Community leaders
- Chambers of Commerce
- Media

these stakeholders on care coordination for the patient's enrolled in the MIH program, another primary reason for communication with external stakeholders is to tell them that you aren't looking to replace or change anything that's already in place and working well. If the patient's need is already being met, there is no need to be addressed.

This small initial project by MedStar helped patients find the resources they needed to manage their healthcare better, thereby reducing the use of emergency services for nonemergency care. The internal goal for this targeted program was to help make ambulance resources more available for higher acuity 9-1-1 calls to enhance MedStar's performance meeting these calls. MedStar's priority was navigating patients to the appropriate healthcare contacts to serve their needs best, whether it was a community or private clinic, a Federally Qualified Health Center (FQHC), home health care, or a physician practice. When you communicate with all of your stakeholders, they'll be more likely to collaborate with you because you will be seen as a resource and not as competition.

Strategic Partnerships

To succeed at creating an MIH program, MedStar had to gather many agencies and personnel around the table. MedStar accomplishes this by creating a Care Coordination Council comprising representatives from the seven area hospitals' case managers and social workers as well as community-based organizations such as the United Way, Meals on Wheels, the Area Agency on Aging, Project Access (a volunteer physician program sponsored by Tarrant County Medical Society[2]), and other community resources. Topics center on specific individual patient needs and how these community health representatives can find solutions to meet those needs.

MedStar actively participates on numerous hospital and community committees and task forces to address issues such as hospital readmissions, preventable emergency department visits, fall prevention, elder abuse prevention, child abuse prevention, motor vehicle crash reduction, end-of-life/palliative care programs, regional STEMI (ST segment elevated myocardial infarction) and stroke councils, medical services for the homeless, and drowning prevention.

MedStar is also represented and has leadership roles in programs such as the University of North Texas' Health Science Center School of Public Health, as a member of the Masters in Healthcare Administration Advisory Board, and Leadership Fort Worth's Healthcare Program Day.

During the first MedStar community meetings with stakeholders, a whiteboard was used to outline issues and needs. The question was asked—what are the difficulties your patients are facing? Everyone contributed, sharing issues such as patient difficulty accessing community clinics or not having enough primary care capacity (the ability to improve the way primary care practices provide care). The whiteboard approach helped people to start thinking about and identifying the gaps that are currently having affecting patient healthcare. By getting stakeholders to talk about their needs, you can position yourself as a potential solution either to meet those needs or to help as a navigator to direct patients to the resources already available in the community. Engaging stakeholders helps them feel that they are part of the solution. When stakeholders are engaged and believe they are part of the process, they'll take ownership in the program and will come up with innovative ideas, suggestions, and recommendations, and they will become advocates and supporters of the programs that you implement.

Remember that MIH and community paramedicine are not one size fits all. In a rural community you may find through the gap analysis that there is a large primary care need because primary care offices may be located far away from the residents. The community and your EMS organization therefore may decide that community paramedics and MIH practitioners need to be able to provide certain types of primary care in a patient's home such as suturing, wound care, administering medications, or other frequent needs. An MIH program in a rural community and one that operates in an urban community might be significantly different.

Your analysis will enable you to target needs and implement the type of MIH program that is appropriate for the areas you serve.

A training program can be developed based on the needs identified in your community. In Fort Worth, it was determined that there was a need to be able to navigate patients to help them get the right care at the right time at the right place (and with the right outcome at the right cost). Linkages needed to be developed between the patient and the resources available in the community. This is the primary difference between an urban MIH model and a rural model. In rural areas MIH practitioners may need to augment primary care or even skilled nursing.

The goal for MedStar is to be viewed as a healthcare provider instead of a method of emergency transportation. Great strides have been made in that direction by transforming the way EMS is delivered. When EMS providers conduct meetings for community health initiatives, they are often viewed as the experts in that arena. Healthcare providers and leaders rely on EMS providers to facilitate solutions, and they succeed when they bring solutions to the table that benefit the patient. Building relationships and a level of trust are critical.

Developing relationships with external stakeholders involves continually reaching out to them to address their needs, and educating them on the services that an innovative MIH provider can bring to improve the healthcare system.

Federal Stakeholders

On the federal level, MIH program leaders have been invited to the halls of Congress and other federal agencies to tell the story of how MIH programs are achieving the IHI Triple Aim.

In the spring of 2013, Gary Wingrove and the North Central EMS Institute in Minnesota hosted a Community Paramedicine briefing. The meeting was held in the offices of the U.S. Senate in our nation's capital. Over 50 representatives from congressional offices and numerous federal agencies attended. During the meeting, they were briefed on the programs and program outcomes in Minnesota; Wake County, NC; Pittsburgh, PA; Eagle County, CO; and Fort Worth, TX. That level of interest from congressional representatives shows the level of attention the MIH transformation is getting in the halls of Congress.

But it's not just the elected officials. In fall 2013, MedStar was requested to participate in the National Academy of Science's Institute of Medicine policy summit addressing the impact of the Affordable Care Act on the emergency care delivery system and emergency preparedness.[3]

MedStar was also invited in June 2012 to present the agency's programs to the Agency for Healthcare Research and Quality (AHRQ),[4] which is the Department of Health and Human Service's healthcare research arm. MedStar and others were invited again to update AHRQ on the MIH programs, as well as brief the agency on the other evolving MIH programs in March 2013 and again in March 2014. The results of these three meetings has been published by the AHRQ on their Healthcare Innovation Exchange.[5]

In March 2014, representatives from the Regional Emergency Medical Services Authority in Reno, NV (awarded a CMS Innovation Award for a community health program[6]); Wake County, NC;

Pittsburgh, PA; and Fort Worth, TX, had the unique opportunity to meet with Patrick Conway, MD, the Chief Medical Officer for CMS. Conway was enthusiastically supportive of the work being done with the MIH programs represented at the meeting and suggested several ways to expand the model in additional communities to increase the number of patients involved in these programs.

Collaboration with Healthcare Accrediting Agencies

As MIH programs mature, it will become increasingly important to engage with stakeholders from healthcare accreditation agencies. Hospitals, home care agencies, skilled nursing facilities, and even payers are subject to accreditation in order to demonstrate compliance with core processes, process improvement strategies, and outcome measures. MIH, and to a large extent, even traditional EMS, is the delivery of healthcare. To fully develop these programs as a quality-driven service delivery model, accreditation from agencies such as the National Committee of Quality Assurance (NCQA), The Joint Commission, or the Utilization Review Accreditation Commission (URAC) will become essential. In March 2014, MedStar met with NCQA and discussed their potential involvement in accreditation for MIH programs. They were very interested in working with the EMS community on accreditation standards for MIH programs such as CHF and high-utilizer programs. URAC has been accrediting disease management and nurse advice services for decades and may be a logical agency to accredit 9-1-1 nurse triage programs. The International Academies of Emergency Dispatch has been accrediting emergency medical dispatch programs and are currently working on accreditation standards for 9-1-1 nurse triage programs as well.

Looking Beyond the Obvious

Sometimes you will discover patient needs that were not even on your radar screen. This was recently the case in Fort Worth, when it was found that some patients referred into the MIH program needed care way beyond the ability of the providers or even a traditional home care agency. In these cases, a solution was found by identifying rehabilitation facilities that had the capacity to care for these patients.

With providers working collaboratively with the patients' physicians, patients were temporarily admitted to these facilities to address a short-term, acute need. Similarly, with providers working collaboratively with the rehab and long-term, acute care facilities, another service gap in the community was discovered: patients who are being discharged from skilled nursing going back to their homes. These patients may have a difficult transition and need additional care, much like the transition from an inpatient hospital stay to home.

When patients have been in a skilled nursing facility for a certain period of time, they rely on care providers and may sometimes lack the confidence in their abilities to live on their own when they return home. MedStar is looking at a model that would fill that gap in care and is taking referrals from facilities or rehab hospitals for patients who they think might have difficulty making that transition or have to be readmitted.

The results of a needs assessment are often invaluable when you involve a variety of stakeholders.

MIH agencies bring valuable perspectives, data, and a mobile workforce that is invaluable to these committee processes. To be successful, be a good support structure and source of knowledge for the physicians, community leaders, and hospitals.

Pearls of WISDOM

Becoming part of the healthcare community and being woven into the fabric of your community should logically start long before you begin the discussion about MIH programs. Start today by surveying the landscape in your community looking for healthcare-related organizations and initiatives with which you can become actively engaged. These could include:

- United Way
- Area Agency on Aging
- A 2-1-1 system (if available in your community)
- Hospital readmission reduction task forces and/or transitions of care committees
- Healthcare for the homeless programs
- Federally Qualified Health Centers
- Local college or university-based healthcare education programs

Are You READY?

- Read the Agency for Healthcare Research and Quality reports on mobile healthcare and community paramedic programs at: http://www.innovations.ahrq.gov/content.aspx?id=3343
- Read the program overview of the REMSA CHIT program at: http://www.remsa-cf.com/community.html
- Learn about the NCQA's accreditation programs at: http://www.ncqa.org/Programs/Accreditation.aspx
- Begin assembling a list of all healthcare and social service providers in your area. Invite the head of each of these agencies to coffee or lunch to learn about their programs and services.

Summary

EMS providers will have to determine the needs of their community. Start by identifying what healthcare services are available in the community and the services that are missing, and then fill that need. Develop relationships and partnerships and become the eyes and ears and hands—the support mechanism—for the improvement of healthcare in the community. The solution will involve training, developing curriculum, and tracking patient data. Mobile integrated healthcare is the solution that enables patients to go where they need to go to get the care they need—the right care at the right cost at the right time.

References

1. National Association of Emergency Medical Technicians. Mobile integrated healthcare and community paramedicine. Available at: http://www.naemt.org/MIH-CP/MIH-CP.aspx. Accessed August 22, 2014.
2. Tarrant County Medical Society. Project Access Tarrant County. Available at: http://www.tcms .org/PATC.aspx. Accessed June 2, 2014.
3. Institute of Medicine. National preparedness impacts of the Affordable Care Act. Available at: http://iom.edu/Activities/PublicHealth/MedPrep/2013-NOV-18.aspx. Accessed June 2, 2014.
4. Agency for Healthcare Research and Quality resources page. Available at: http://www.ahrq.gov/. Accessed June 2, 2014.
5. U.S. Department of Health and Human Services. Trained paramedics provide ongoing support to frequent 9-1-1 callers, reducing use of ambulance and emergency department services. Available at: http://innovations.ahrq.gov/content.aspx?id=3343. Accessed June 2, 2014.
6. Regional Emergency Medical Services Authority. Community health programs. Available at: http://www.nursehealthline.com/partner. Accessed June 2, 2014.

5

Program Development

To be truly successful, mobile integrated healthcare programs must be mobile (focused on navigating patients, even those in remote areas, to the appropriate healthcare resources), integrated (with hospitals and others in the community), and patient centered (focusing on providing healthcare). The development of your program should be based on the needs assessment of your community and involves working with all of the stakeholders to create a program that fills the gaps in your healthcare system.

The New Program Model

The old model of an EMS team response with transport of the patient to an emergency department is a vertically fragmented system approach that is not patient centered. This system is being replaced by an innovative new approach. MIH programs offer your community a patient-centered, horizontal systems approach that is connected and delivers comprehensive care for the patient in collaboration with other healthcare providers in the community. There are two basic models for MIH programs. One is the primary care replacement model, and the other is the urban model.

The primary care model may include the provision of primary care such as suturing, medication administration, wound care, and long-term in-home care management if home healthcare is unavailable. The urban model is essentially patient navigation that involves directing patients to the most appropriate healthcare resources already available in the community.

In Chicago, one mobile integrated healthcare program focuses on preventing hospital readmissions among patients with congestive heart failure (CHF). The participating EMS agency is Skokie-based Medical Express (MedEx.) Their collaborative organizations include home health providers, universities, and hospitals, including the University of Chicago Medicine; Health Resource Solutions (HRS); Allscripts, which provides an integrated electronic health record; and HomeScript Pharmacy, which delivers medications to patients.

Here's how it works: patients with CHF who are discharged from the University of Chicago health system are transported home by MedEx. HRS provides ongoing education and care as needed, with EMS available for emergencies. MedEx and other mobile integrated healthcare partners are available for patients through a 24-hour call center. The professionals who answer the calls focus on navigating patients to the appropriate MIH partners such as cardiologists, primary care physicians, nurses, social workers, home health providers, therapists, advanced practice nurses, and pharmacists. Each person plays a role, and initiating program development involves awareness and education.

Understanding the Regulatory Environment

The way your new mobile integrated healthcare program operates within the community may be different than how programs operate in another city or state, depending on your state laws. When you consult with organizations, officials, and EMS programs in other communities, make sure they understand their own regulatory landscape. The regulations that apply in Chicago may not apply in New York.

Texas is a delegated practice state, which means that there is no state protocol or scope of practice for emergency medical services. The local medical director makes the determination of which skills and medical treatment the EMS providers deliver and the training that they receive. EMS systems can perform a variety of procedures in Texas, as long as the medical director authorizes the proper training. For example, if a medical director wants paramedics to perform intubation, the paramedics operating under the medical director's license will be authorized to perform intubation. Without complete support of the medical director, an MIH program will not be successful. Know the scope of service that your program is allowed to practice. Know your regulatory environment, and establish relationships to help make your program a success.

MedStar providers have had success performing home patient assessments, interfacing with the patient's primary care physician, educating patients on medications and healthy habits, and helping patients manage chronic diseases. Providers even administer Lasix or morphine without the need for patient transport to the emergency department. Providers have given what is considered extended care in the patient's home under the umbrella of MedStar's successful mobile integrated healthcare program.

How many times have you responded to an unconscious patient with diabetes, and, once you administer glucose IV, the patient wakes up and is completely competent and doesn't want to be transported. On the other extreme, patients in cardiac arrest may require that you perform ALS for 20 or 30 minutes with no change in condition. More and more in progressive EMS systems, resuscitation will be terminated and the patient will not be transported to the hospital.

The basis for MIH is nothing really new—EMS providers have been doing it for years—assessment, treatment, and referral. Interestingly, many years ago the Centers for Medicare and Medicaid Services (CMS) agreed to pay EMS providers for the assessment and treatment without transport of one medical condition: cardiac arrest. CMS likely did the math for this scenario and found out when cardiac arrest patients were transported for the ability to bill for the service, the downstream cost to CMS was astronomical. So instead, CMS allowed EMS to get paid for treatment without transport for cardiac arrest victims.

Providing assessments, providing proper medical treatments, and offering patient education for patients who are not transported to the hospital are not outside the scope of practice for EMTs and paramedics in Texas. However, in some communities, if you are administering antibiotics or if you are performing advanced treatments in the home such as suturing, it is considered an expanded scope of practice, by definition, and requires regulatory approval. Understand your regulatory environment before you initiate those programs in your local community.

Key Positions in Program Development

The Medical Director

Mobile integrated healthcare is exactly what the name implies. It is healthcare integrated into the community using mobile resources, and the emphasis is on providing the appropriate healthcare rather than transporting patients in the old "you call, we haul" model. The program medical director is one of the most important leaders in this entire transformation because the medical director is involved in everything—provider selection, provider training, patient selection, and quality assurance.

MedStar's medical director during the evolution of the MIH program was a licensed paramedic and an emergency department physician part time in the community. He understood the nuances of delivering emergency medical services and how they can play a larger role in the healthcare system. The EMS medical director in your community may also be a physician, and that relationship is invaluable to establish. The medical director has to be 100% committed—not just involved—in the program. When MedStar's medical director talks about traditional EMS, he talks about making 300 house calls a day using MedStar's EMTs and paramedics. Another MedStar team member, the associate medical director, is a private practice physician and part of the North Texas Specialty Physicians group (NTSP). He connected MedStar with NTSP to create MedStar's first agreement for payment for implementing some of these programs in the mobile setting.

Build relationships with your physician groups. They are invaluable in helping you execute important healthcare integration strategies.

EMS Practitioners vs. MIH Practitioners

When traditional emergency medical services personnel transition to an MIH program, there are several things to keep in mind. First, in a successful MIH program you're looking for the clinician and practitioner personality—the individual who has skills and abilities to nurture people, communicate effectively, and perform follow-up. The MIH practitioner educates patients to take care of themselves and teaches them, through patience and practical advice, how to manage their disease and thereby reduce the potential for hospital readmission.

Most EMTs and paramedics thrive on the adrenaline of excitement and immediate problem solving. They are by definition technicians—they typically see an event, react to it, and provide treatment following a specific protocol. An average time to transport the patient to an emergency department is 30–45 minutes. It could, however, be less than 25 minutes.

An MIH practitioner requires personal skills in addition to those typically provided by EMTs and paramedics. Identify your MIH care providers not only by their current abilities and excellence in achieving performance standards, but by the future role they'll perform. The MIH role is different because it establishes long-term relationships within the community. Identify paramedics who understand the bigger picture of patient care within the healthcare system. MIH providers connect with patients to effectively communicate and strategize about their health care. This provider will be able to fit all of the pieces of the puzzle together to provide patient education and navigation to the right place at the right time.

The paramedics who take 30 or 45 minutes on the scene of a call because they are educating the patient and family are the providers best suited for the new role in mobile integrated healthcare! They are nurturing during on-site visits, strengthening relationships, and understanding patient needs and then fulfilling them.

The traditional paramedic personality is sometimes referred to as the Johnny and Roy syndrome, based on the television series *Emergency!* in the 1970s, because the characters were all about saving lives. Every call was an adrenaline rush—they rescued people trapped in cars, had at least one cardiac arrest every episode, and never seemed to have repeated calls for patients suffering from alcohol abuse. The show educated Americans about the EMS system in an era when there weren't many providers in the nation. However, that is not a realistic portrayal of what EMS does every day. The traditional paramedic is adept at short-term interaction with patients and transport to an emergency department and then moving on to another call.

Although the traditional paramedic role is still needed in the EMS community, the MIH role requires the ability to build relationships over longer periods of time. In MIH, you'll need providers who want to make a difference in the patient's health over the long term—providers who will spend an hour or two at the homes of patients during each visit, helping them learn about the disease process and understand ways they can take better care of themselves. This type of paramedic wants to see that patient change over time, which is different than providing the type of EMS care of the past.

Solid critical thinking, or being able to recognize problems and find a workable means for meeting those problems, is another trait that is an asset to have as an MIH practitioner. The ideal practitioner understands the connection between a step toward better health that the patient takes now and what that might mean to the patient tomorrow or the next day. This practitioner has a good understanding of the body systems and the pharmacologic needs and other interventions that may be involved over time. MIH takes critical thinking to the next level.

For example, a patient who frequently falls may need to be referred to a program that can go into the home and install grab rails or secure carpeting. There are programs that help make homes safe for elderly patients, and there are other programs to assist with psychological needs. MIH practitioners recognize these issues and act as critical thinking problem solvers to help find solutions for these patients. If providers see a patient who falls regularly in the home because of stacks of magazines and papers and old trash or other objects, they might find a specialist to help organize the home or they may refer the patient to a local mental or behavioral health agency. If a patient needs counseling, the MIH practitioner can help coordinate a solution.

The education that I was provided was more in-depth and beneficial than any doctor or hospital ever provided to me, especially the weekly visits of someone who genuinely concerned about my well-being. Instead of constantly going to the hospital and being processed by very busy staff, I was treated like a friend by the paramedics. I was able to use the education to empower myself to make the changes I needed to make. I learned from John the importance of hydration, what certain temperatures do to your muscles, and since the stomach is a muscle, this was very vital. I learned the warning signs, dangers, and effects of high blood pressure from Marissa. These factors helped me use my body like a machine—what to do, when to do it, and what to look out for. And from both of these individuals, I learned the signs and symptoms of an actual physical addiction to pain medication. Until someone took the time to explain these signs and symptoms to me, in a way I could relate and in my environment of comfort, I had no idea that I was addicted to pain medicine. Mine was not an addiction to pain medicine I bought on the street—it was an addiction to the medicine the doctor gives to you because they truly believe it will help you.

Once I realized I was addicted, I was able to reach deep inside my spirit and wean myself off pain medicine completely. I haven't had pain medicine in almost 4 months, not even over the counter.

Antoine Hall
MedStar MIH patient

Other solutions for elderly patients or patients with diabetes to have a regular source of healthy food may involve programs such as Meals on Wheels. Meals on Wheels can ensure that patients receive at least one good meal a day, which helps prevent hypoglycemia and a trip to the emergency department.

In most communities there are a myriad of agencies that can help patients and help coordinate the care they need, to make sure the patient is able to manage their disease process and take care of themselves out of the hospital setting.

Provider Selection and Training

As mentioned earlier, depending on the role that MIH is going to play in your local community, you may have the opportunity to use a variety of different types of providers. For example, if you're implementing only basic community paramedicine, you may need to use paramedics to be able to achieve all you need to do in that program. However, there may be patients who would benefit from care provided by an EMT or emergency medical responder organizations in the system. You may also find that some of the programs that you develop may require other types of trained and qualified personnel. For example you may need a team of nurse practitioners, physician's assistants, or in some cases even physicians to fill gaps in services that were determined during your needs assessment process. Provider selection depends on the program that you're implementing and the roles you need to fill.

In one model at Mesa Fire Department in Arizona, a nurse practitioner is paired with a fire department captain/paramedic to respond to low-acuity calls. In your community, if you're providing occupational health or physician services, physicians need to be available on call.

Throughout this book the emphasis has been that MIH programs are locally driven and therefore need to meet a gap that exists or serve as a bridge to appropriate care in the local healthcare system. Right now it is a challenge to write any type of national curriculum that will work in northwestern Montana yet also work in the New York City. Although some core components may be fairly similar, most of the training that the EMTs, paramedics, or other staff is going to need must be specifically tailored for a local healthcare system.

This process of transitioning the nation from EMS to mobile integrated healthcare is often centered on reducing costs and hospital readmissions and in training paramedics in the skills patients most need in the community. All EMS systems have loyalty program members, also known as frequent fliers, people who frequently call 9-1-1 for nonemergency care and are transported to the emergency department. If your community has identified that reducing the number of low-acuity calls to 9-1-1 is a goal of the MIH program, you'll need a specific training module, localized with your community stakeholders, in order to effectively train your personnel to help patients navigate to the most appropriate healthcare resource (**Table 5-1**).

Table 5-1 Sample Module: Module 3. Clinical Medicine Overview for Mobile Integrated Healthcare

Module Description

(6 Hours)

Recommended Target Audience

Practitioners with a minimum of 2 years as EMT/Paramedic or higher

Prerequisite

Base knowledge of entry-level paramedicine according to the National Emergency Medicine Services Educational Standard curriculum; MIH program Modules 1 and 2

Module Goal

To convey the clinical knowledge to perform the clinical role of a mobile healthcare practitioner

Module Objectives

Upon conclusion of this module, the student will be able to:

1. Explain the base knowledge of anatomy and physiology required to perform the clinical role of a mobile healthcare practitioner.
2. Explain the influences of culture, environment, and psychosocial aspects on the physiological disease progression and management for individuals experiencing impaired health states.
3. Differentiate the patient encounter of traditional EMS and MIH programs.
4. Explain the impact of commonly prescribed and over-the-counter medications and the importance of medication reconciliation and compliance in the MIH program environment.
5. Analyze lab values, and integrate these values into patient assessment and integration into clinical decisions.
6. Identify the types, operations, and complications of common medical devices used in outpatient settings.

Training for paramedics who will be working with frequent 9-1-1 users in the community should include home visits as well as rotations in community clinics and hands-on training with patients with behavioral health issues. Rotations in the local homeless shelters or housing projects as well as visits to behavioral health centers will help paramedics understand what to expect. A majority of EMS loyalty program members have behavioral health issues. Working in a behavioral health environment will give the paramedic a valuable perspective on caring for patients with behavioral problems.

Other modules that may be included in the training program might be congestive heart failure readmission prevention, diabetes and asthma management, hospice programs, and primary care interventions.

The results of the community needs assessment will determine the role you need to fill, which will drive the type of training you plan and implement. Regardless of the type of training, it is important to include the professionals who will be interacting with those providers. For example, in an EMS loyalty program, the education involves the local case managers and local ED physicians. You'll also want to involve public health authorities, homeless shelter staff, and others.

If you're planning to implement a congestive heart failure module, you would conduct congestive heart failure training and include the local cardiologists and CHF clinics in your community. To familiarize your staff with the expectations of the local healthcare community, conduct training and attend rotations in clinics so relationships can be built. See how providers in the community want their patients cared for in the field. Patient-focused collaboration becomes easier when you develop relationships with stakeholders and begin to communicate with them on a first-name basis.

In a congestive heart failure program, the paramedic in the home helps the patient manage the disease and will facilitate the coordination of care with the patient's primary care network and the other systems that are in place to assist the patient with long-term management of the disease process. The goal of MIH is to help patients manage their own care outside of the hospital and reduce the number of 9-1-1 calls by offering them more appropriate, accessible options for treatment. These options may include referring patients to a number of community-based organizations that are designed to meet some of their physical or psychosocial needs.

The Care Coordination Council

One thing you may want to consider is developing a care coordination council, which is a group that has been meeting for years at MedStar in order to strengthen relationships with case managers and participants from all of the hospitals, along with other community partners.

The council may include members of your own local agencies and healthcare organizations such as Meals on Wheels, the Area Agency on Aging, the behavioral health association, rehab hospitals, and anyone else who is involved in caring for a particular patient or group of patients. The meeting facilitates positive sharing and communication about how to better serve the patients in the program. Ideas focus on helping patients navigate the healthcare system by coordinating care with other first response or co-responders in your community.

Coordination of patient care among EMS providers, hospitals, and others in the healthcare system enables an accurate, true understanding of the utilization of the system in which the patient's care can be monitored and coordinated properly. If, for example, a frequent 9-1-1 user has been transported to two different emergency departments during 1 month where he received medication, your collaboration and communication with others in the system help you better understand the patient's condition and situation and how to effectively respond.

Quality Assurance

As you begin to create your MIH program, it's important to build in a process of quality assurance. Quality assurance involves activities and programs intended to ensure or improve the quality of care in a medical program. The concept includes the assessment or evaluation of the quality of care; identification of problems or shortcomings in the delivery of care; designing activities to overcome these deficiencies; and follow-up monitoring to ensure effectiveness of corrective steps. Earlier chapters discussed not being afraid to make mistakes and incorporating that philosophy into your training along with a strong process of quality assurance.

A culture of openness fosters good communication and sets expectations internally. When a new program is implemented, all the participants are learning. It is valuable to build in a process for the free exchange of ideas, questions, and feedback. Training should also include feedback from cardiologists, nephrologists, and other specialists who can discuss various disease processes and drug interactions, such as specific drug interactions with the cardiac system or the impact of certain medications on the renal system. Outside experts can accelerate the learning process and prepare the team for situations they might not ordinarily experience.

Quality assurance plays a pivotal role in your MIH program as you grow. The program progresses with an ongoing learn-as-you-go approach and continuing education on a real-time basis every time an MIH practitioner calls a physician or interacts with a case worker. Interaction with a patient's primary physician, for example, to discuss medication, treatment, or follow-up, educates providers in developing a patient care plan. When new patients enter your program, your team will be developing the patient care plan and initiating communication with the patient's primary care physician. Training in specific communication skills and collaboration is vital. As relationships with patients develop over time, practitioners in the field learn more about the disease process or multiple comorbidities of their patients and how to provide long-term care. It is educational for the paramedic and fosters a lot of questions!

Ongoing training may include follow-up meetings with healthcare practitioners and physicians' groups. Biweekly meetings with all of the MIH practitioners are held by MedStar. The team shares and discusses information on specific patients, medications, medical devices, and other patient treatments and programs, with the goal of continual improvement in the program. These meetings also provide an opportunity to review the outcomes of some of the patients with the medical director to improve patient care and review other patient scenarios and similar disease processes for additional learning.

The *integrated* part of mobile integrated health care means coordinating and integrating a patient's care with the rest of the healthcare system, which is something that needs to be done for every patient. Paramedics in the field need to be appropriately trained and able to communicate clearly with a variety of professionals and patients.

Lessons Learned

Program development requires resiliency and the ability to evolve the programs as you go. The first version of MedStar's congestive heart failure program did not include strong primary care physician (PCP) commitment or a diuretic protocol. Consequently, MIH practitioners taught patients how to recognize the warning signs of disease exacerbation, but they did not have the ability to intervene or make follow-up appointments for the patients. This lead to an increase in the number of ED visits. Refinement of the program involved ensuring commitment from PCPs and, in return, a diuretic protocol. Since then, the program has reduced the number of ED visits and readmissions in the enrolled patients by 75%.

Are You **READY?**

- Go to the National Association of EMT's catalog of MIH programs and review the types of programs currently operating at http://www.naemt.org/MIH-CP/MIH-CPResources.aspx.

- Review the National Association of State EMS Officials' MIH Committee mission, vision, and meeting minutes at https://www.nasemso.org/Projects/MobileIntegratedHealth/index.asp.

- Meet with your internal stakeholders (service chief, medical director, labor union (if applicable), and begin discussions on the possible selection criteria for MIH providers. This should be based on the gaps identified by your community needs assessment that can potentially be filled by your MIH program.

Summary

As you can see, there are many parts to implementing an effective MIH program. The MedStar MIH program has been a major factor in preventing hospital readmissions for specific chronic diseases such as COPD, diabetes, and CHF. These diseases can be managed by the patient with the appropriate education, awareness, and specific daily steps and healthy habits. The MedStar program has been designed with the patient in mind, and the MIH providers are working to teach and educate other community EMS providers how to do the same.

The foundation is to work collaboratively with your local community stakeholders to develop a program designed to bridge identified gaps or needs in your community. Then, develop a training program that involves the stakeholders and MIH practitioners, select the right practitioners, and provide ongoing care coordination, education, and quality assurance. A "no" mentality just won't work in the MIH program. You need people who say "yes" and can find solutions to problems.

6

Types of Mobile Integrated Healthcare Programs

Change is constant, and when the circumstances around you change, people are left with a choice—to adapt or be left behind. The environment created by the rapid shifts in our healthcare system provides an unprecedented opportunity for emergency medical services (EMS) to become more of a part of the overall healthcare delivery system. A mobile integrated health (MIH) program is an excellent way for EMS to increase their role in the system. As mentioned previously, the success or failure of your MIH program will depend, in large part, on the program's ability to meet a local gap in the healthcare services available in your community.

This chapter will discuss the basic types of MIH models being followed, as well as some specific program design components of the MedStar MIH program.

MIH Models

In general, MIH models can be categorized as a *primary care* or a *patient navigation* model. Primary care models are often found in rural or frontier areas when the closest primary care may be hours away. In these models, paramedics or other midlevel practitioners may actually perform primary care such as suturing, catheter placement or maintenance, prescribing or administering medications in consultation with a physician a great distance away, or other similar types of services. The following sections highlight examples of primary care models.

Examples of Primary Care Models

Eagle County Paramedics, Eagle County, Colorado

Program goals and methods include:

- Ensure all patients have a medical home.

- Reduce rehospitalizations by 50%.

- Enhance injury prevention versus potential costs associated with no prevention.

- Enhance number of vaccinations given and public health visits.

- Provide postdischarge follow-up.

- Provide primary care follow-up.

- Provide school-based health.

- Provide injury prevention.

- Provide public health services.

- Provide social services adult protection visits.

- Provide in-home lab services.

North Memorial Medical Center, Minneapolis, Minnesota
Program goals and methods include:

- MIH practitioners are staffed in three primary clinics in the north Minneapolis area.

- See 12–14 patients per 12-hour shift.

- Assigned patients by a clinic coordinator

- Primary care focused

- Patients need to have a care plan or be in a medical home.

- Medical home and care plan avoids duplication of service.

- Focus is on patients with chronic disease, with a heavy emphasis on patients with diabetes.

- Assistance with wound management

- All lab work completed is on site.

- Tracks frequent ED utilization with follow-up

Patient Navigation Models
The following sections highlight examples of patient navigation models.

Regional Emergency Medical Services, Reno, NV
Program goals and methods include:

- Create new care and referral pathways that ensure patients who have entered the 9-1-1 emergency medical services system with urgent low-acuity medical conditions receive the safest, most appropriate levels of quality care.

- Postdischarge patients with conditions such as congestive heart failure will receive in-home follow-up care.

- The Nurse Health Line provides 24/7 assessment, clinical education, triage, and referral to healthcare and community services via a nonemergency nurse health line available to all Washoe County residents regardless of insurance status.

- Community health paramedics are specially trained to perform in-home delegated tasks to improve the transition of care from hospital to home, perform point-of-care lab tests, and improve care plan adherence.

- The Ambulance Transport Alternatives program provides alternative pathways of care for 9-1-1 patients, including transport of psychiatric patients directly to the mental health hospital, transport of inebriated patients directly to the detoxification center, and transport of 9-1-1 patients with low-acuity medical conditions to urgent care centers and clinics.

Center for Emergency Medicine – Western Pennsylvania

Program goals and methods include:

- Improve patient outcomes and experience of care.

- Reduce preventable ED visits and hospitalizations.

- Primary focus is on familiar faces and vulnerable patients.

- Regional service delivery model with referrals from 45 EMS agencies and 15 hospitals in Allegheny County (Pittsburgh and surrounding communities)

- Complete psychosocial assessment by a community paramedic, who then serves as patient navigator, patient advocate, and health coach to get the patient enrolled in applicable social service agencies

The MedStar Model

MedStar decided early on to be an innovative organization and leverage the changes coming in the healthcare industry. By developing an MIH program, MedStar found solutions to existing healthcare issues in the community and at the same time a way to prepare for the future. One of the many positive outcomes of this change included the new relationships and connections that have strengthened employee satisfaction and improved MedStar's position in the community, earning the trust and recognition of the healthcare system.

The First Step: The EMS Loyalty Program

MedStar's first venture down the road of MIH was trying to help individuals who were frequent users of 9-1-1. These persons are called the EMS loyalty program members. The program was initiated in July 2009 and primarily driven internally to reduce the low-acuity call load that was occurring on a regular basis. An overview of the program is shown in **Figure 6-1**. The goal of the program was to make more resources available to improve MedStar's response time performance. The program began by using a light-duty paramedic who knew the system and the loyalty program members well.

Program Overview – High Utilizer 9-1-1/Emergency Department Patients

Background

MedStar Mobile Healthcare has been operating a Community Health Program (CHP) using Mobile Healthcare Practitioners (MHP) since July 2009. Patients who have graduated from the CHP have experienced an 84.3% reduction in emergency department (ED) use for the 12 months post-graduation compared to the 12 months pre-enrollment. MedStar works together with the patient and numerous healthcare and community-based providers to reduce the incidence of preventable ambulance responses and ED visits.

Program Components

Patient Education & Scheduled Home Visits:

An enrolled patient receives a series of home visits conducted by a specially trained MedStar Mobile Healthcare Practitioner (MHP). These home visits are designed to:

1. Educate the patient and patient's family on the appropriate ways to manage their healthcare needs. The patient is also assessed for possible enrollment in various healthcare and community-based programs to help meet the patient's clinical, social and/or behavioral health needs. This includes:

   a. Medication compliance
   b. Healthy lifestyle changes
   c. Nutritional support
   d. Home environment/safety needs
   e. Behavioral health support

2. Educate the patient how to utilize their primary/specialty care network to help manage their medical needs. This includes:

   a. When to call for an appointment
   b. How to call for an appointment
   c. Important information to share with care providers
   d. How to utilize transportation services

During the intake visit, the patient is also asked to assess their own health status using the EQ-5D-3L process by EuroQol.

Unscheduled Home Visits:

The patient is provided a 10-digit, non-emergency access number for the MedStar Mobile Healthcare Provider in the event they would like a phone consultation or an unscheduled home visit between scheduled visits.

9-1-1 Responses:

Enrolled patients are tracked in MedStar's 9-1-1 computer aided dispatch (CAD) program. In the event of a 9-1-1 call to the residence, the normal EMS system response is initiated, but the MHP is also dispatched to the scene. Once on-scene, the MHP may be able to intervene and prevent an unnecessary ambulance trip to the emergency department by employing the use of the alternative protocols available to the patient enrolled in this program.

MedStar Mobile Healthcare ◆ 551 E. Berry Street ◆ Fort Worth, TX 76110
www.medstar911.org

Figure 6-1 MedStar program guidelines. (*Continues*)

Record Keeping:

Patients enrolled in the program have a continual electronic medical record (EMR) that allows all care providers mobile access to the patient's entire course of assessments and treatments during enrollment, including care notes, vital signs, ECG tracings and treatments initiated. These records can be electronically provided to any care giver with access to a fax or email account.

Care Coordination:

MedStar hosts monthly meetings with all case workers, community service agencies and other care providers to review the program and enrolled patients in an effort to help meet any needs of the enrolled patients and to improve program resource coordination.

Graduation:

After the patient has demonstrated the ability to better manage their healthcare needs, the patient is graduated from the program, provided a graduation certificate, a patient satisfaction survey and the patient is asked to re-assess their own health status using the EQ-5D-3L process by EuroQol. This data is tracked to help measure program effectiveness and identify area of potential improvement.

Figure 6-1 MedStar program guidelines. (*Continued*)

A report from the MedStar business office detailed patients who called 9-1-1 multiple times and then ranked them by frequency. We discovered that 21 patients called 9-1-1 fifteen or more times in 90 days. These patients were considered the *executive platinum-level* members of the EMS loyalty program! The initial 21 patients who were evaluated had 2,000 9-1-1 responses during the previous year; if the number of unnecessary calls could be reduced, a slowdown in the growth of personnel hiring would occur and MedStar would be able to meet the response time desires in the community.

The 21 patients who were frequent users were contacted and asked whether they would be interested in enrolling in a new innovative program designed to help them find better resources for their medical care to reduce the number of 9-1-1 calls and emergency department visits. Eighteen patients agreed to enroll in the program, and MedStar MIH practitioners began working with them on a regular basis. Patient participants signed a consent form that not only allowed practitioners to schedule proactive home visits with them, but also provided HIPAA authorization in order to share the patient's information with other providers to coordinate care in an effort to reduce the reliance on 9-1-1 and the emergency department system for primary medical care (**Figure 6-2**). Home visits, visits at the homeless shelter, or visits at the street corner in a tent city for the homeless were done. Providers did whatever it took to educate patients and connect them with resources in the community to meet their needs and to determine the leading cause of their 9-1-1 use as the primary source of medical care. The reasons were found to be diverse.

One patient called 9-1-1 regularly because he did not know how to enroll in the county's indigent care program. He had been told by the emergency department case managers and other professionals that he needed to enroll in the program, but he could not accomplish the enrollment process. Like so many things in the healthcare system, navigating the enrollment process to become eligible to receive services from the county's indigent care program was very complex. MedStar therefore learned the enrollment process and helped patients enroll in a program that gives them access to multiple clinics and primary care physicians in the community.

Another patient had a primary care physician and clinics available to him, but he did not drive and was afraid to take the bus. He therefore used 9-1-1 to be transported to the emergency room to receive primary care. MedStar took the time to ride with the patient on the bus, show him where the bus stops were, and where the transfer station was, giving him greater freedom and the resources he needed to manage his own healthcare. He learned how to use the public transportation system to be able to access his primary care.

Another patient was calling 9-1-1 almost every other week on a Friday because her pain medication would run out and she needed to go to the hospital for a refill. By doing frequent home visits with this patient, counting her pills, and watching her take her medications on schedule, it was quickly discovered that her family members were stealing her medications and selling them on the street. So for the cost of a $19.50 drug safe, the patient was able to make sure that her pain medication was not stolen and she had enough pills to manage her condition. She no longer needed to make a call to 9-1-1 to refill her medications.

MOBILE HEALTHCARE PROGRAM
Referral Form

Person Making Referral: _____   Date of Referral: ___/___/___

Phone :(____) _____-_____   Fax :(____) _____-_____   E-Mail:_____

Affiliation to Patient: ❑ Hospital Caseworker   ❑ Social Worker   ❑ Primary Care Physician

❑ Name of Referral Agency: _____

❑ Funding Source: _____

_____   DOB: ___/___/___   Age: _____   Sex: ____
Patient Name

_____   (____) _____-_____
Address   Phone

_____   _____   (____) _____-_____
Emergency Contact   Relationship   Phone

_____   (____) _____-_____
Primary Care Physician   Phone

_____   (____) _____-_____
Cardiologist   Phone

_____   (____) _____-_____
Pulmonologist   Phone

_____   (____) _____-_____
Endocrinologist   Phone

_____   (____) _____-_____
Other   Phone

Primary Medical Condition: _____

(Please attach most recent copy of Facesheet and H&P with any discharge instruction then fax to 817-632-0530)

MedStar MHP Referral Form.doc   Page 1 of 5

Figure 6-2 Sample referral form. (*Continues*)

MOBILE HEALTHCARE PROGRAM
Type of Service Requested

Services to be provided at:

❑ Place of Residence   ❑ Place of Employment

❑ Other Location: _____

Blood Pressure Screening/Monitoring
Please describe frequency of monitoring and any special instructions:

BGL Screening/Monitoring
Please describe frequency of monitoring and any special instructions:

ECG Tracing
Please describe frequency and duration of monitoring, where a copy of the ECG tracing should be sent and any special instructions:

Fall – Risk Assessment
Please describe any specific concerns regarding the space to be assessed

Immunization/Vaccination:_____ **(type)**
Please indicate type of vaccine, where it is to be obtained, and site/route preference and general administration instructions

MedStar MHP v2.doc   MEDSTAR   Page 2 of 5

Figure 6-2 Sample referral form. (*Continues*)

MOBILE HEALTHCARE PROGRAM
Type of Service Requested

Prescription Drug Compliance Monitoring
  Indicate the name, type, dose and frequency of Rx, and frequency of compliance monitoring

General Assessment/Social Interaction
  Indicate the frequency and general type of social interaction that may help the patient feel safe and secure in their home environment

Weight Monitoring
  Please describe frequency of monitoring and any special instructions

Other Assessments or Interventions:
  Please describe frequency of monitoring and any special instructions

Reviewed by: _____   **Date:** ___/___/___
        MedStar Medical Director/Community Health Coordinator

MedStar MHP v2.doc   Page 3 of 5

Figure 6-2 Sample referral form. (*Continues*)

MedStar Mobile Healthcare
COMMUNITY HEALTH PROGRAM (CHP)
CONSENT FOR CARE

I, the patient/patient's legal representative, hereby grant permission to MedStar, to perform such examinations and medical and therapeutic procedures professionally deemed necessary or advisable for my/the patient's diagnosis and treatment.

I acknowledge that MedStar is primarily an emergency medical service based healthcare provider and that paramedics and emergency medical technicians authorized by the EMS Medical Director will be providing the care rendered.

CONSENT FOR RELEASE OF INFORMATION

I hereby authorize the MedStar to release:

1.   Any or all of my/the patient's medical information from and to the referring physicians, physician assistants, health care providers, including a public health nurse, or home health agency referral, insurance companies, and other third party sponsors to facilitate health care, processing of claims, audit of payments for hospitalization and/or treatment, and to facilitate overall assessment of the CHP effectiveness. I understand that the information released may include records in these areas: HIV/AIDS, sexually transmitted disease, mental health treatment, and drug and alcohol abuse treatment.

2.   Basic patient information regarding date and time of appointment(s) to family members (parents, spouses, adult children, guardians), and caregivers.

PRIVACY NOTICE

We keep a record of the health care services we provide you/the patient in either a printed or an Electronic Medical Record. You may ask us to see a copy of that record. You may also ask us to correct that record. We will not disclose your record to others unless you direct us to do so or unless the law authorizes or compels us to do so.

These consents may be revoked at any time except to the extent already relied upon. Unless earlier revoked by written notice filed with MedStar, these consents shall expire three years after the date of last treatment.

I have read, understood and agreed with the above information:

_____   ___/___/___
Patient's Signature   Date

_____   ___/___/___
Print Name   DOB

_____   ___/___/___
Witness   Date

_____
Print Name

(If Patient is under 18 years of age, or the patient has been deemed incompetent to make decision regarding their healthcare services, a parent, or legal guardian must read Release and complete information below)

_____   ___/___/___   ___/___/___
Parent/Legal Guardian's Signature   Date   DOB

_____   _____
Print Name   Relationship

(In the event Patient, or the Parent/Legal Guardian in the case of a minor patient, refuses to sign this form, this fact should be noted on the refusal form and the form placed in Patient's file.)

MedStar MHP v2.doc   **MEDSTAR**   Page 4 of 5

Figure 6-2 Sample referral form. (*Continues*)

REFUSAL OF MEDICAL CARE
ACKNOWLEDGEMENT
MedStar Community Health Program

I, _____, acknowledge that I have been offered services under the MedStar
         Print Name
Community Health Program (MedStar CHP) and hereby acknowledge my refusal of medical/health care, treatment and/or
services under this program.

I further acknowledge that I have been informed of the risks involved as a consequence of my refusal, and on behalf of
myself, my family, heirs, and personal representatives, I release MedStar, its participating providers, municipalities,
officers, representatives, independent contractors, agents, and employees from all present and future responsibility,
liability, claims, demands, actions and causes of action whatsoever, whether known or unknown, foreseeable or
unforeseeable, arising out of or related to any loss, damage, expense, illness, injury or aggravation of illness or injury
(including death) that I may sustain or incur as a direct or indirect result of my refusal of medical/health care, treatment
and/or services under the MedStar CHP.

I agree that the laws of the State of Texas govern this Release, and the venue for any legal proceeding that may arise
concerning my refusal of medical treatment is Tarrant County, Texas.

_____   ___/___/___
Patient's Signature   Date

_____   ___/___/___
Print Name   DOB

_____   ___/___/___
Witness   Date

_____
Print Name

**(If Patient is under 18 years of age, or the patient has been deemed incompetent to make decision regarding their
healthcare services, a parent, or legal guardian must read Release and complete information below)**

_____   ___/___/___   ___/___/___
Parent/Legal Guardian's Signature   Date   DOB

_____   _____
Print Name   Relationship

(In the event Patient, or the Parent/Legal Guardian in the case of a minor patient, refuses to sign this form, this fact
should be noted on this form and the form placed in Patient's file.)

MedStar MHP v2.doc   MEDSTAR   Page 5 of 5

Figure 6-2 Sample referral form. (*Continued*)

Another patient who had congestive heart failure with an ejection fraction of 30 was calling 9-1-1 frequently in the late afternoon or early evening. Upon assessing this patient's home environment, it was noted that he lived in a third-floor walk-up apartment in an apartment complex. He said that when he arrived home from work it would take him 30 minutes to walk up to the third floor because he would climb the first flight of stairs and then wait at the landing to catch his breath. After climbing the second set of stairs he would stop again to catch his breath. Often, by the time he got to the top of the third floor he was having such difficulty breathing that he needed to call 9-1-1 and receive acute care in the emergency department. As a solution, MIH paramedics were able to speak with the building manager and have the patient relocated to a first-floor apartment so he wouldn't have to climb up several flights of stairs to get to his apartment. His use of 9-1-1 decreased because he was able to easily reach his apartment despite his medical condition.

These scenarios represent only a few examples of the situations that MedStar found once patients were enrolled in the EMS loyalty program. MedStar provided personalized solutions for the patients and recognized that often they did not need healthcare services—they needed to be connected to resources that were already available to them in the community. In every community this lack of knowledge exists, and many patients are unaware of or unable to access services in order to help meet their medical or social needs.

Patients are also registered in MedStar's 9-1-1 computer-aided dispatch system so when they do call 9-1-1, MedStar can send the normal emergency medical services response based on the Advanced Medical Priority Dispatch System's (AMPDS) response determinate, or an MIH practitioner can respond to the call to see whether the patient can be navigated to a more appropriate care setting. The key to the success of this community health program is that a select number of patients have voluntarily enrolled, and they are being managed by a core group of paramedics who know these patients well, who see them on a regular basis, and who know their medical history and social and mental health needs. In general, MedStar MIH practitioners work with these patients for 60 to 90 days in an effort to help them change their access points for primary medical needs. If after 60 to 90 days the patient demonstrates that he or she is unable or unwilling to change the frequent use of 9-1-1 for nonemergency care, the patient is transitioned into MedStar's system abuser status.

When patients are designated as system abusers, MIH practitioners no longer do proactive home visits. MedStar does keep these patients registered in the 9-1-1 computer-aided dispatch system so when they do call 9-1-1, in addition to the regular response determined by the AMPDS®, an MIH practitioner responds to the scene. Once an MIH practitioner arrives on scene, a patient assessment can be completed. Again, this is a core group of patients being managed by a core group of paramedics, so they know each other well. If the MIH practitioner determines that the patient should receive medical care from a setting other than a hospital emergency department, the practitioner can contact the medical director or associate medical director by phone from the scene and discuss and confirm the approach to care. In most cases, the medical director knows this patient well. The medical director and MIH practitioner are able to discuss the most appropriate source of medical care necessary for the patient. The medical director may recommend that patient be transported to the emergency department. By definition, these patients generally have medical needs, comorbidities, or behavioral health issues that may require acute care. However, the medical director may determine the patient's condition can be treated more appropriately by a primary care physician, clinic, or other healthcare setting. The patient is provided with a taxi voucher, a bus pass, or other means to carry out the recommendation provided by the medical director.

The MIH approach to patient care is not about denying the patient service. The goal of MIH is to navigate patients to the right service and teach them how to use their primary care system. MIH attempts to provide patients with a medical home that can follow up on their short-term and long-term care.

After MedStar's MIH program was implemented, a 48% reduction was seen in 9-1-1 use by the initial 18 patients in the first 90 days. That's a remarkably reduced call volume. But the rewards extended beyond a simple reduction in the number of calls. The patients were receiving better care, making better decisions, and feeling more empowered.

The success of MedStar's first step allowed more resources to be available to respond to higher acuity calls; the patient satisfaction for the EMS loyalty program was very high. MedStar knew that the MIH program would bring additional value to the healthcare system in our community. MedStar connects patients to resources that are already available. This program, the first community health program, was initially designed to connect patients to resources that were already available in the community without duplicating services and to utilize those resources on behalf of the patient's health more effectively—the hallmark of all of the MIH programs that have been developed.

The Stakeholder Response

After the initial pilot program, the next step was to assemble all of the healthcare stakeholders to discuss the opportunities that are available as a community to bring MIH to patients who were frequently using the 9-1-1 and emergency department system. The community needs assessment was completed by meeting with staff from the hospitals, the case managers, United Way, the mental health associations, and all of the stakeholders that were previously identified.

The stakeholders were asked several questions to understand what their needs were: What resources might be available? Did they feel that MedStar's role in bridging that gap would be valuable not only to the patient but to their agencies? As discussed earlier, because of the collaboration and the relationships that MedStar had with many of the healthcare system stakeholders in Fort Worth, the audience was very receptive. The stakeholders were willing to help MedStar develop a more formalized program that addressed frequent 9-1-1 users in the community.

At the same time, MedStar's medical director wanted to introduce a specialized level of paramedic response to the high-acuity, low-frequency 9-1-1 calls. For EMS systems that may use the Medical Priority Consultant's AMPDS®, these calls would be the ECHO calls, such as cardiac arrest, severe difficulty breathing with a changing level of consciousness, and other potentially life-threatening medical emergencies.

Training Programs for MIH Practitioners
Critical Care Transport Program

MedStar knew that revenue would need to be generated early to offset some of the costs of providing a dedicated mobile integrated healthcare resource for the community. A critical care transport (CCT) program could potentially provide that revenue, but it was a program that MedStar had not pursued simply because of the lack of resources to meet the agency's 9-1-1 demand. As a result, another provider in the service area was authorized to provide CCT. MedStar believed that if they were able to provide CCT, and do it effectively, the revenue from the CCT program would be able to offset some of the cost of providing the mobile integrated healthcare program. From this idea, a business plan was put together that assembled all of the anticipated costs—from personnel to training, equipment, and vehicles. The costs were then combined with the potential revenue generated from the critical care program, which could potentially eliminate some of the field positions because of the reduced number of calls that were coming into the system.

MedStar's medical director and associate medical director went to the emergency physicians advisory board (EPAB) with the concept of dedicated single paramedic units managing high acuity, low-frequency calls and providing CCT. The EPAB wholeheartedly endorsed and supported the creation of the program. The ED physicians understood that EMS and emergency department resources were not being used effectively and that initiating a CCT program to offset the costs of an MIH program was an important step toward better utilization of resources and patient care. With the full support of the healthcare stakeholders and MedStar's medical control authority and ambulance authority board, the process of selecting providers to participate in CCT training began. At the time there was no training program available so MedStar developed one.

The critical care transport class helped MIH practitioners care for the EMS loyalty program members because of the additional pathophysiology and the advanced assessment skills that they learned. Two additional course components were added. The first was MedStar's community health program education class, which teaches MIH practitioners the resources that are available in the community, how to access them, and how to enroll patients in them. Experts were brought in to teach practitioners how to enroll patients in the public health indigent care program. They were taught about behavioral health from the mental health and mental retardation association of the county. They were taught about the services provided through the United Way, Meals On Wheels, and other programs in the community. This education was done in the classroom and clinical setting. Providers participated in rideouts with the mental health mobile crisis outreach team. They spent time with the medical directors in the emergency department and other clinical settings to see how low-acuity patients were treated in an emergency. They also were taught the advanced skills necessary to manage a cardiac arrest more effectively, which included therapeutic hypothermia and grief counseling. MedStar has an assertive cessation-of-resuscitation policy. To cease resuscitation in the field, everyone at the scene needs to agree to cessation—not only the MedStar crew but the first responders and the family members. MIH practitioners therefore were taught how to address bereavement and provided grief counseling.

MedStar's education program teaches the staff about the patient-treatment process for cardiac arrest and resuscitation, as well as how to care for the family members. The paramedics communicate openly with family members, involving them in the resuscitation, and explain to them everything that is going on at the scene. The paramedics may cease resuscitative efforts in the patient's home. They became well versed in explaining to family members that all of the care their loved one would normally receive in the emergency department is being provided right there, and transport to the hospital is unnecessary.

When the training program was completed, the MIH practitioners graduated and began using a single paramedic MIH unit in the field 24 hours a day, 7 days a week, to treat frequent patient users and respond to ECHO calls to provide an additional resource on scene for the responding units.

Congestive Heart Failure Program

As mentioned in an earlier chapter, congestive heart failure (CHF) is one of the top killers in the United States and creates chronic emergency department visits and hospital admissions because of the nature of the disease. The emergency physicians advisory board received patient data bimonthly from the CHF program.

In June 2010, several months after the community health program was initiated, MedStar was approached by a large cardiology group in the Fort Worth area with the idea of reducing preventable readmissions. They shared that it was likely Medicare would soon begin penalizing hospitals and physicians for unnecessary 30-day readmission rates for congestive heart failure. They asked MedStar to work with them on a program to see whether the 30-day readmission rate for patients with congestive heart failure could be reduced. MedStar worked collaboratively with the medical control authority and the cardiology group to put together an initial demonstration project for the prevention of congestive heart failure readmission.

The early part of the program involved case managers referring patients who were at risk for potential readmission within 30 days. MIH practitioners would do proactive home visits to those patients to educate them on their discharge instructions because often when patients are being discharged from the hospital they are unable to take in all of the discharge instructions. However, once patients are home, sitting at *their* kitchen table with *their* spouse or other loved ones, they are ready to understand the instructions. In the home environment MIH practitioners can clearly educate discharged patients about why pizza, sodas, or potato chips are not good to eat to manage their disease, or why they need to weigh themselves daily and record their weight. A medication inventory is also done to make sure that patients have the correct prescriptions, there are no duplicates, and that all of the prescriptions have been filled. A home environmental assessment can determine whether there are risks of falling or other dangers that require resources.

MIH practitioners mitigate risk and then register those patients in the 9-1-1 computer-aided dispatch system in case they need to call 9-1-1. Practitioners provide patients with the 10-digit non-emergency number to call so they don't have to call 9-1-1, and a baseline assessment is performed. A baseline 12-lead ECG is obtained, given to the patient, and attached to the patient's electronic medical record. Patients have baseline lab values available to them through the MIH program and IStat blood analyzer, so if necessary, practitioners can provide point-of-care testing to determine the patient's metabolic state to help the patient's primary care physician determine the best course of treatment for the patient.

Observation Admission Avoidance Program

Observational admissions are a significant focus of the Centers for Medicaid and Medicare Services (CMS) due to a 69% increase in admissions over the last 5 years. An observational admission is an admission that occurs in the emergency department when patients are not admitted as inpatients, but not discharged from the emergency department. These patients are typically held for 24 or 48 hours in the emergency room or some other department in the hospital in an outpatient status because they are awaiting lab results or other tests or require general observation. The typical scenario for an observational admission maybe an elderly patient who enters the emergency department after a fall. The patient's CT scan is normal, MRI is normal, and blood work is relatively normal, but the emergency department physician may not feel comfortable sending the patient home without knowing more about the patient's clinical condition or home environment. These patients typically have a follow-up appointment scheduled with their primary care physician or specialist for the next day or on a Monday if the visit occurred over the weekend.

There are many challenges when the patient is held under observational admission. First, the resources in the emergency department are being used for patients who are being observed. Second, observational admissions are billed at a higher rate to CMS or another payer because the admission does not result in a diagnosis-related group (DRG) payment for an inpatient stay. Third, the patients typically have a higher deductible or copayment for outpatient observation. Finally, because the patient was not admitted to the hospital, the patient is not eligible for skilled nursing or rehab benefits if they are needed. A significant financial burden may result for the patient, the family, and in some cases even the payer.

The observation admission avoidance program was brought to MedStar by the associate medical director, who is one of the partners in North Texas Specialty Physicians (NTSP). NTSP was part of an accountable care organization (ACO) in partnership with a large hospital system in the community. These two entities partnered to develop one of the pioneer ACOs under CMS.

The executive director of the Independent Practice Association (IPA) told MedStar that each observational admission cost the ACO approximately $5,400, so their goal was to reduce the admission by $5,400 and make it safe for the patient to be at home by providing the resources and in-home visits necessary during the time between the emergency department visit and the follow-up doctor visit. MedStar worked collaboratively to put together a program for the ACO.

VOICES OF EXPERIENCE

Being homeless I couldn't always take my medicine because I couldn't get to a bathroom in time, so I filled up and couldn't breathe. You guys helped me learn how to monitor myself and take care of myself even though I was homeless. If it wasn't for you guys working with everyone I would still be homeless, but now I am in a nursing home and not homeless anymore. If it wasn't for what MedStar did for me I would probably be in the hospital again or maybe even dead. I wish I could do something to show you all how happy I am for what you did. I am very thankful for everything you guys did for me.

Larry Erickson
MedStar MIH patient

The emergency department physician or the case manager working in the emergency department recommends the patient as a good fit for the MedStar MIH program under the observational admission avoidance program. If the patient seems to qualify based on the emergency department physician's assessment, the case manager calls MedStar. MedStar arrives at the emergency department within 60 minutes to have a brief meeting with the emergency department physician and the patient who is being sent home to determine the focus of the patient's care during the 24–48 hour enrollment. After the patient returns home, an MIH practitioner visits within a few hours. On this follow-up visit, a practitioner not only reviews the discharge instructions with the patient, but a home assessment is done to determine whether changes in the patient's environment need to be recommended. Specifically, if the patient is a fall risk and has four cats that move faster than the patient, loose carpeting in the home, or no grab rails, there is room for improvement to make the home safer. Are there other dietary issues that need to be addressed? Are there other environmental hazards that might need to be discussed with other community partners to improve the safety of the home? Patients in the program are given the 10-digit nonemergency number to contact MedStar's 24/7 call center if they feel uncomfortable or if they would like to have an episodic visit before their follow-up appointment with the physician.

The next day, or whenever the patient's appointment is scheduled, MedStar can share the patient's information from the visit either through an electronic health information exchange or by using the call center triage nurse to call the physician's office and review the documentation. The information can be sent electronically or in print to the nurse in the physician's office in time for the patient's follow-up appointment. The triage nurse can also confirm the appointment and if necessary assist with making any transportation arrangements to ensure the patient does not miss the follow up appointment. Everything is connected!

Since MedStar started the observation admission avoidance program, 87 patients have been enrolled, and only 3 patients required another emergency department visit prior to the follow-up physician appointment, and the second visit was unrelated to the first stay. Not only does the program provide a safe environment for the patient by doing an in-home assessment during the visit, but MIH practitioners can also be available if the patient has another unrecognized medical condition. They can make sure the patient is navigated to the appropriate resources, which in one case was a visit to the emergency department.

The ACO did an analysis of the first 11 patients enrolled in the program and found on average a savings of $7,800 per patient—quite a bit more than what they thought they would be under this program. Patients therefore continue to be enrolled in this successful program.

Hospice Revocation Avoidance Program

MedStar was approached by a local division of a national hospice agency who had heard about the successes of the community health program through mobile integrated healthcare. A hospice per-day patient fee averages between $150 and $300. When the patient is admitted to inpatient hospice, which is care usually provided in a hospice facility or designated part of a nursing home, the rate is slightly higher. Once the patient is enrolled in hospice, the hospice agency is responsible for paying all of the patient's hospice-related medical expenses. For example, if a patient receiving hospice care at home needs to be taken by ambulance to the emergency department for a hospice-related event, the ambulance charge, the emergency department charge, and all of the charges that go along with the care received by the patient for the episode of care are billed to the hospice agency. The hospice agency collaborated with MedStar in an effort to reduce the expenses for hospice patients while maintaining palliative care.

Under the hospice enrollment, the patient and the family members have agreed they want palliative care provided to make the patient comfortable until death. It is not unusual, however, for families to activate the 9-1-1 system when the patient is near death and becomes restless, which typically results in an emergency ambulance response, along with the fire department, and transport to the emergency department or, in some cases, perhaps even resuscitation efforts. Often, patients or family members are unable to produce do-not-resuscitate documentation or other paperwork, and resuscitative efforts are initiated.

Caring for patients in hospice and their family members is very stressful and difficult for the patient, the family, and the responding agencies. When someone calls 9-1-1 for a hospice patient, typically the patient is too difficult to be taken care of at home, and the caller wants "everything done" so the emergency medical services system is activated. During this situation, there is a significant risk that the family may elect to voluntarily disenroll the patient from the hospice program. If a patient voluntarily disenrolls from hospice, the financial impact on the hospice agency is double-edged. First the agency loses the revenue that they would normally receive for the per-patient care day fee and the length of stay that the patient remains in hospice. Second, the hospice agency is responsible for paying for the medical expenses for that hospice-related event prior to the voluntary disenrollment paperwork being filed. Patients suffer because their initial desires for end-of-life care are not met. In general, when a voluntary disenrollment occurs, it's a mess for the patient, the family members, the caregivers, and the hospice agency.

Patients can also be disenrolled from hospice by the hospice agency. The hospice agency has the ability under the guidelines to involuntarily disenroll or revoke a patient's hospice status if the patient or the patient's family is not compliant with the program and creating medical expenses that would not usually be necessary under the normal palliative care course of care. In this case, the hospice agency elects to revoke the patient's hospice status and therefore reduce the risk of additional medical expenses, which again is not an ideal scenario for the patient, the family members, or the hospice agency.

The hospice agency uses a specialized risk assessment tool for determining which patients or families are at high risk for voluntarily disenrolling from hospice. The hospice program refers those patients to MedStar's MIH program, which responds in a few key ways. First, practitioners and the hospice nurse visit the patient's home to explain the partnership between the hospice agency and the mobile integrated healthcare agency. This visit includes reminding the patient and family members that the hospice nurse is the primary point of contact for their needs. However, if for any reason they're unable to reach their hospice nurse, the patient has access to MedStar's 10-digit number to call for access to care in an emergency. If a call is made, an MIH practitioner visits the home and cares for the patient's needs until the hospice nurse is reached.

In the event of a 9-1-1 call, the hospice nurse registered in the computer-aided dispatch system is notified that an emergency response is being made to the house. The registration ensures continuity of care in the MIH program and has the phone number for the hospice nurse who is caring for the patient. A quick response time may help avoid involuntary disenrollment.

If the 9-1-1 response was related to the patient's hospice condition, the MIH practitioner can remind the family that the patient's desire was palliative care at home. Hospice patients will typically have a comfort pack of medications that have been given to them by the hospice agency. The MIH practitioner can assist the patient in taking medications such as morphine or other analgesics to help the patient become more comfortable. The MIH practitioner can also provide counseling for the family and reassurance, reminding the family that the patient desired to transition in the home setting. During the care process, the family's permission can be obtained to relieve the first responders and allow the ambulance to leave. MIH practitioners stay with the family members and the patient until the hospice nurse arrives to ensure the patient's comfort and help keep the patient in the hospice program.

In the event that the 9-1-1 response was not related to the patient's course of care for hospice, the patient is transported to the emergency department. For example, a patient with congestive heart failure who is receiving at-home hospice care who has fallen and received an injury can be transferred by ambulance to the emergency department without any potential risk of hospice revocation or any expense to the hospice agency.

If in consultation with the family members and the patient's hospice nurse it is determined that the patient requires *inpatient* hospice care, the MIH practitioner and hospice nurse can counsel the family members and make arrangements for the patient to be transferred from the home hospice setting to an inpatient hospice setting at a facility designated by the hospice agency. Therefore, it is a hospice plan of care transport without running the risk of a voluntary disenrollment or a revocation of hospice status.

Since MedStar began the partnership with hospice, 149 patients have been enrolled into the program. There were 11 revocations of voluntary disenrollment—remember that these patients were identified by the hospice agency as families at *high risk*—so a 10% revocation rate is significantly better than the 30% or 40% or higher voluntary disenrollment percentage that the hospice agency was expecting.

9-1-1 Nurse Triage Program

An earlier chapter discussed that 36.6% of MedStar's 9-1-1 requests do not result in an emergency response. Many people call 9-1-1 for medical or trauma conditions that could more appropriately be cared for in ways other than an ambulance trip to an emergency department. The 9-1-1 nurse triage program helps navigate callers for very low-acuity medical or trauma conditions to settings such as a primary care physician office, dental office, urgent care facility, or even self-care at home.

Requests for a 9-1-1 response are initially categorized by MedStar's certified emergency medical dispatch (EMD) call takers using the AMPDS® by Medical Priority Consultants (**Figures 6-3** and **6-4**). MedStar's 9-1-1 call center is one of only 144 centers in the nation to be designated as an Accredited Center of Excellence (ACE) by the International Academies of Emergency Dispatch (IAED).

These protocols and the response configurations assigned to them are developed by an international medical board of specialists based upon millions of patient encounters. The protocols and response configurations assigned to the call types are developed and approved based on MedStar's medical control authority, the emergency physicians advisory board (EPAB).

The 9-1-1 nurse triage system, officially called the emergency communications nurse system (ECNS), can be implemented by call centers that are ACE accredited to ensure the highest level of compliance with EMD protocols. The ECNS relies on the nurse's education, training, and experience to assess patients using computer-based algorithms that have been developed by the IAED and used extensively in the National Health Service in the United Kingdom. EPAB reviewed these algorithms and have approved them for use in the MedStar 9-1-1 call center.

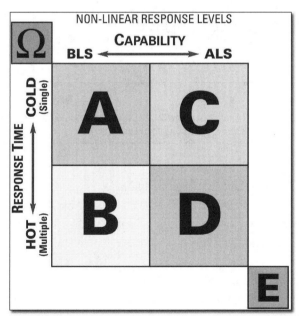

LEVELS	#	DETERMINANT DESCRIPTORS ➔ E	CODES	RESPONSES
D	1	**Not** breathing (**after** Key Questioning)	12-D-1	Agency Determined Responses Here
	2	**CONTINUOUS** or **MULTIPLE** seizures	12-D-2	
	3	**AGONAL/INEFFECTIVE BREATHING**	12-D-3	
	4	Effective breathing **not** verified ≥ 35	12-D-4	

Figure 6-3 Categories of response levels.

Non-linear Response Level Matrix. The MPDS v13 protocols. © 1978-2014 International Academies of Emergency Dispatch. Reproduced with permission.

Baseline Response Example

All actual response assignments are decided by local Medical Control and EMS Administration

Level	Response	Mode
ECHO	Closest Apparatus–Any (includes Truck Companies, HAZMAT, or on-air staff)	HOT
DELTA	Closest BLS Engine Paramedic Ambulance	HOT HOT
CHARLIE	Paramedic Ambulance	COLD
BRAVO	Closest BLS Engine BLS Ambulance (alone HOT if closest)	HOT COLD
ALPHA	BLS Ambulance	COLD
OMEGA	Referral or Alternate Care	

*Note: This is **not** to be considered the Academy's official recommendation for Baseline Responses.

Figure 6-4 Response example.

Example of one system's baseline response choices for each level. Other systems may not do it this way. Principles of EMD, 5th edition, ©1988-2014 International Academy of Emergency Medical Dispatch. Reproduced with permission.

Based on caller information, calls are categorized from lowest priority (OMEGA) to highest priority (ECHO). Low-acuity calls that are approved by EPAB to be eligible for the nurse triage system are transferred to the nurse in MedStar's call center using a warm handoff. The caller is advised by the 9-1-1 call taker that based on the condition explained by phone, the patient may benefit from MedStar's in-house nurse to determine whether there is a safe alternative to an ambulance to the emergency department. While the caller is on the line with the EMD, the EMD adds the nurse onto the call (the caller is never placed on hold), the EMD introduces the caller to the nurse and summarizes the caller's situation. The nurse then stays on the line while the EMD drops off. The nurse uses his or her education and experience, with the ECNS decision support algorithms, to more fully assess the patient's condition and determine a locus of care most appropriate for the patient. The locus of care categories are as follows:

Emergency ambulance response: The nurse notifies the MedStar dispatcher to send an ambulance for an emergency response. MedStar personnel remain with the patient as long as possible during the response.

Nonemergency ambulance response: A nonemergency ambulance response is initiated and will respond under normal road conditions without lights or sirens; the response may take up to 20 minutes.

Mobile healthcare practitioner response: A specially trained MedStar MIH practitioner responds within the hour to further assist the patient.

Patient needs an emergency department: The patient requires assessment at an emergency department; however, the patient does not require an ambulance to get there. The nurse may arrange transportation for the patient if the patient does not have a transportation source.

Urgent care center: The patient should be seen at an urgent care center for further evaluation. The nurse may arrange transportation for the patient if the patient does not have a transportation source.

Contact primary care physician: The patient is advised to contact his or her primary care physician (PCP) for further advice and management. In many cases, the nurse will call the PCP's office with the caller on the phone.

Self-care: The patient is advised how to care for his or her illness or injury at home, without necessarily the need for follow-up care. The nurse will call back in a specified period of time to check in on the patient.

Contact dentist: The patient is advised to contact the dentist for further advice and management. In many cases, the nurse will call the dentist's office with the caller on the phone.

Contact poison control: The nurse calls poison control with the caller on the phone to seek advice.

Contact obstetrician: The patient is advised to contact her OB/GYN for further advice and management. In many cases, the nurse will call the OB/GYN office with the caller on the phone.

Contact public health department: From the symptoms reported, the nurse needs to contact the local health department. The patient's primary care physician should be contacted with any further questions.

Contact mental health team: The patient may benefit from contact with the mental health advisor or crisis team. This contact is done with the caller on the phone.

In all cases in which the patient disposition was something other than an ambulance to the emergency department, the nurse follows up by calling the patient within 24 hours. This follow-up is a requirement of the program and designed to determine how the patient is doing, whether or not the patient followed the advice, and to ensure everything is going well. Approximately one week after initial contact, the patient is contacted by MedStar's quality improvement team and asked a series of questions regarding MedStar's customer service. The answers to these questions are tracked and reported on periodically.

Between June 2012 and May 2014, 1,620 calls from 9-1-1 were referred to the on-duty triage nurse. Of these, 658 calls received a disposition other than an ambulance to an emergency department. Interestingly, the experiential data from patient interviews reveals that on a Likert scale of 1–5, with 5 being the most satisfied, the average score for patients who received an alternate disposition was 4.7; 85.8% of the patients indicated their condition got better, and 93.4% said that speaking with the nurse helped. Even more interestingly, of the patients who called 9-1-1 and received something other than an ambulance trip to an ED, 76.8% of the patients who responded to the customer experience survey stated the way their call was handled was the way it should have been handled.

The program works!

Patient Empowerment

The goal of the MIH program is to empower patients to manage their own healthcare and to teach them how to live a healthier lifestyle with their medical conditions. What are the allowable foods on their diet? What other things do they need to do? MIH practitioners don't tell patients what they cannot do; they educate patients about what they *can* do. How do they access their cardiologist or their primary care physician for the best healthcare possible? Practitioners also teach patients how to ask questions and how to report on conditions or situations that might be going on at home with their weight and medication. Patients become better, more informed patients for the physicians who are managing the disease process; these patients are able to identify early on when they begin to decompensate and warrant care.

Early in the program, MedStar realized that the relationship with the primary care physician or the cardiologist had not been adequately developed, and practitioners had a difficult time scheduling appointments for patients in a reasonable timeframe. As a result, when patients recognized that they were beginning to decompensate, they would call MedStar or their primary care physician. Either way, a call would be placed to the patient's primary care physician indicating the need for a timely appointment. Often, the appointment could not be made, and practitioners were unable to navigate the backdoor to the physician's office to make the appointment. In fact, in some cases, the receptionist at the primary care physician's office would tell the MIH practitioner or the patient to call MedStar! As a result, patients were transported to the emergency department for treatment when timely appointments could not be made.

Consequently, the first outcomes of this program resulted in an increase in emergency department visits. Patients had a decrease in the actual admissions, however, because they were identified early as decompensating—before they got into more serious trouble. Patients needed less intervention in the emergency department; however, MedStar's goal was to avoid ambulance transfers for the visit to the emergency department.

Phase 2 of the program to engage primary care physicians with MIH practitioners evolved during a cardiology group meeting when one of the cardiologists said,

> You know, if you guys see a patient with CHF and that patient ends up in the emergency room, the emergency room physician is going to diurese the patient in the ER and send them home. Or worse, they're going to diurese the patient in the emergency department and admit them. If we could just diurese them in a setting that doesn't require the emergency department, we can avoid the ED visit and the potential admission. So how about having mobile healthcare paramedics diurese these patients at home?

Farhan Ali, MD, a cardiologist on the emergency physicians advisory board and some of the cardiology groups were approached with the concept of MIH practitioners being able to assist in the treatment of these patients. The MedStar medical director and assistant director were supportive of MIH practitioners performing diuresis in a patient's home. MedStar therefore worked collaboratively with the community and drafted a new in-home diuresis protocol. To complete a diuresis protocol, the MIH practitioner needed to have access to the patient's primary care physician to schedule an immediate appointment if in-home diuresis was to be performed. MedStar needed enough MIH practitioners in the field to be able to do a timely follow-up on those patients once a diuretic had been administered. A clinical plan and an operational plan therefore were developed.

The clinical plan involved enrollment criteria—to be eligible for this protocol, the physician needed to be committed to receive calls from MIH practitioners in the field to help determine the right course of care for the patient. The physician needed to commit to making a follow-up appointment immediately available for that patient in the office to avoid an emergency department visit.

MedStar needed to provide a second resource in the field so if the patient needed to have a follow-up within 4 hours, practitioners were available to provide that care. A second MIH paramedic was placed on duty Monday through Friday, 10 am to 8 pm, to help ensure that immediate follow-ups could be performed. MedStar also needed to provide additional clinical assessment information to the physician and verify that the correct patients were receiving diuretics. An IStat blood analyzer was purchased to administer point-of-care testing for BUN, creatinine, potassium, and other values to check the patient's kidney functioning before in-home diuresis begins.

Once MedStar began using the in-home diuresis protocol, a significant difference in patient readmission and ED visits was noted. With committed physicians and effective interventions that could be provided in the home, MedStar was able to reduce the frequency of readmissions and even emergency department visits by 96% in this target population.

Expanded Role vs. Expanded Scope of Practice

Everything that this book has discussed so far involves routine care that paramedics normally provide. Even administering Lasix or nitrates or performing 12 leads or certain lab analyses are not outside the normal scope of practice for paramedics. The only difference is that the definitive care provided does not require ambulance transport or an emergency department visit—the care is coordinated by an MIH practitioner with the patient's primary care physician or cardiologist. Paramedics have an expanded role, not an expanded scope of practice.

When the MIH program first started, MedStar referred to the paramedics in the program as *advanced practice paramedics*, but the title wasn't a good fit because the paramedics were doing very little advanced practice, but they were practicing an important additional role. The title was therefore changed to mobile healthcare paramedic, and then later changed to mobile healthcare practitioner, or MIH practitioner, because the healthcare providers could be EMTs, paramedics, RNs, NPs, PAs, or even MDs.

The Data

Managing patients differently through MIH has proven very beneficial for the patient and all of the stakeholders in the MedStar community. As of April 30, 2014, 340 patients had been enrolled into the community health program, and there was enough data on 88 of those patients to be able to analyze their behavior change—12 months of data before enrollment into the system and 12 months of data after graduation, or when the patient completed the program.

MedStar does not include data on patients who moved out of the area or who stopped calling 9-1-1 for reasons other than a change in behavior. A 48% reduction in 9-1-1 use by patients enrolled in the program was noted, but more importantly, after graduation, patients sustained a reduction in 9-1-1 use by 86%.

Providing Value

As an EMS provider, it's possible you've asked yourself, "How do I really bring value to the patient and the community? What exactly is the value of an EMS provider?" The term *value* not only refers to the value to the patient, but also to the *payer*, the person who writes the check to allow MedStar or any other agency to pay employees, keep ambulances on the street, and keep lights on in the building. Focusing on value in your organization allows you to provide even greater value and resources to those you serve. Providing value can position you and your organization as the go-to expert and leader in the marketplace.

The new healthcare environment has transformed what's possible for EMS and has given those in the profession the opportunity to create new relationships and connections they might not have had in the past. The value of EMS to patients, therefore, can be derived from something as needed and necessary as pain management. EMS providers prevent further injury to patients by giving them safe transport to the hospital; but from the payer's perspective, what have EMS providers done to demonstrate value to the payer? Can something better be done for patients?

Can anyone point to a study in any peer-reviewed publication that indicates that a patient's outcome at the hospital was different because that patient was transported by ambulance to the hospital? Was their length of stay shorter or their overall cost of care less? The outcome from the payer's perspective would be the same whether the patient was transported by taxi, a stranger, a bystander, or a family member.

Many years ago the National Association of EMTs began teaching prehospital trauma life support (PHTLS). The program arose from a study in New York City in the 1980s that looked at modes of transportation to the hospital emergency department for patients who experienced penetrating trauma. The study compared four modes of transportation and patient survival—ALS ambulance, BLS ambulance, police car, and taxicab. Of those four modes of transportation, the highest survival rate for penetrating trauma was the taxicab. The police car came in second. The ALS ambulance had the worst rate of patient survival of the four modes of transportation. This type of finding was reinforced by a 2013 study[1] conducted in Philadelphia that reviewed survival rates for penetrating trauma and concluded once again that patients with penetrating trauma transported by police car had the highest survival rate. Why? It is because paramedics have been trained to do everything possible for the patient on the scene of a call. A patient with penetrating trauma requires an operating room, however, not a 20-minute time on scene for treatment. The PHTLS program was designed to train paramedics for these scenarios—providing value to the patient.

Many of you may remember some of the innovative treatments over the last decade or two—MAST trousers or EGTAs or rotating tourniquets. These devices were thought to bring value to patients. However, over time it was found that they did not improve the patient's outcome. Determining the value of certain treatments continues to be a challenge today. Some may say, however, that the advances in treatment for ST elevation MI (STEMI) and stroke by rapid assessment and rapid preparation of the receiving hospital have improved patient outcomes.

Remember from the value-based purchasing scenario described in an earlier chapter that significant improvements have been made in the treatment of congestive heart failure because you can transport patients from the moment of onset or the symptom onset to a percutaneous coronary intervention (PCI) center and have them quickly receive a PCI. In some cases this intervention may prevent patients from having a myocardial infarction by potentially increasing their cardiac function. The same could be said for the current processes for treating acute stroke, or brain attack. For the other 95% of calls that EMS providers respond to, however, it would be difficult to demonstrate clinical or even financial value based on the treatment given to those patients.

MedStar's MIH program has been able to demonstrate significant clinical improvement and financial benefit by navigating patients effectively through the healthcare system and changing the entire dynamic behind what happens to patients when they call 9-1-1 and their referral and or treatment at a receiving facility. The concept of patient navigation is ensuring the right resource at the right time to the right patient for the right outcome and at the right cost.

Over the years MedStar worked to resolve challenging issues such as hospital diversion, unified protocols, first-response interaction, and quality assurance. The emergency physicians advisory board was well-positioned and had a relationship not only with all of the hospitals but also with MedStar so that mobile integrated healthcare programs could be implemented to bring more value to the patient and the community.

It works!

Lessons Learned

Don't assume what your community needs! MedStar was asked recently by an EMS agency to help them develop an MIH program for their local community focusing on CHF readmission prevention. After development of the program, the agency presented the plan to the hospital only to find that the hospital actually was concerned less about the CHF readmission rate than they were about the rate of unnecessary ED visits due to diabetes. Thankfully, the EMS agency was able to shift gears and quickly develop a proposal for following up on diabetic patients. Make sure you engage your stakeholders early in the process of what gaps you can fill in the healthcare delivery system.

Are You **READY?**

■ Go to MedStar's website, and review the types of programs they are currently operating. http://www.medstar9-1-1.org/community-health-program

■ Request a copy of the community paramedic handbook at http://www.communityparamedic.org/Program-Handbook

■ Read *Beyond 9-1-1: State and Community Strategies for Expanding the Primary Care Role of First Responders* published by the National Conference of State Legislatures at http://www.ncsl.org/research/health/expanding-the-primary-care-role-of-first-responder.aspx

Summary

The MIH programs implemented collaboratively with healthcare system stakeholders based on defined community need fill a gap in the local healthcare system. You need to engage your local stakeholders to determine gaps in your local community that you can effectively fill to improve patient healthcare. Developing or implementing these programs in "tubes of excellence" (previously referred to as "silos") may not achieve the goal the community needs. Implementing programs that patients, payers, and other stakeholders perceive as valuable will help ensure long-term sustainability for the programs.

Reference

1.   Avril T. Police transport a good bet for shooting victims, study finds. January 9, 2014. *Philadelphia Inquirer*. Available at: http://articles.philly.com/2014-01-09/news/45995105_1_gunshot-victims-police-car-shooting-victims. Accessed June 23, 2014.

Data Tracking and Performance Measures

Data collection and tracking are important components of a mobile integrated healthcare program. The benefits of the mobile integrated healthcare program, the methodologies behind the implementation, and the importance of connecting with the community have been discussed. When your program is up and running, however, you'll want to create and implement an effective process for tracking and performance.

Data collection for a mobile integrated healthcare program is significantly different than the data collection for traditional emergency medical services (**Table 7-1**). Traditional EMS looks at process and productivity measures such as response times, task times, cardiac arrest survival rates, cost per unit hour, cost per transport, revenue per transport, and sometimes, but not always, patient satisfaction. In the MIH environment, the stakeholders and customers review data measures based on the previously discussed IHI Triple Aim methodology. Specifically, patient outcome is the focus—the patient's experience of care and the cost of providing that care.

Focusing on process measures does not allow EMS agencies to realize the potential value that can be brought to the healthcare delivery system. To demonstrate value, agencies need to transition to the MIH measures shown in Table 7-1. Change is inevitable.

A recent example of the pressure that will be placed on ambulance and EMS agencies was published in the *New York Times*.[1] Some of the more notable quotes follow.

> *Thirty years ago ambulance rides were generally provided free of charge, underwritten by taxpayers as a municipal service or provided by volunteers. Today, like the rest of the healthcare system in the United States, most ambulance services operate as businesses and contribute to America's escalating medical bills. Often, they are a high-cost prequel to expensive emergency room visits.*

> *Although ambulances are often requested by a bystander or summoned by 9-1-1 dispatchers, they are almost always billed to the patient involved. And the charges, as well as insurance coverage, range widely, from zero to tens of thousands of dollars.*

> *In such a fragmented system, it is hard to know how much high-priced ambulance transport contributes nationally to America's $2.7 trillion health care bill. And total out-of-pocket expenditures by individuals are hard to tally.*

Table 7-1 Comparison of Data Collection

Traditional EMS	Mobile Healthcare
Episode based	Patient based
Focused on an individual encounter with one patient	Focused on multiple encounters with the same patient
Electronic patient care record	Electronic medical record
Patient cared for, incident closed and billed	Continual record to append *all* encounters with the same patient
Limited additional documentation	Multiple additional records
Possible 12L ECG attached	Hospital discharge summary/instructions
	Medication inventory
	Serial vital signs
	Serial lab values
	Assessment of health status
	Patient satisfaction survey
	Provider satisfaction survey
	Environmental/home assessment
	Referral agencies contacted
Cost of service delivery	Value of service delivery
For budgeting and billing purposes	Improvement in health status
	Expenditures avoided
	Resources saved
Episode-based billing	Outcome-based billing
Bill for patient transport	Billing based on improved patient outcome
One patient encounter, one bill	Monthly roster billing
	Patient enrollment billing
Patient experience and satisfaction	Patient experience and satisfaction
Mailed survey cards	Independently managed
Internally received and reviewed	Sent and received by outside agency
Based on agency determined questions	Based on HCAHPS* format used by healthcare partners
Not benchmarked against other agencies	Benchmarked against other agencies

*HCAHPS indicates the Hospital Consumer Assessment of Healthcare Providers and Systems. The HCAHPS provides a core set of questions that can be used with hospital- or agency-specific questions for surveys.

But Medicare, the insurance program for the elderly, does tabulate its numbers and has become alarmed at its fast-rising expenditures for ambulance rides: nearly $6 billion a year, up from just $2 billion in 2002.

That is true even though Medicare's fixed payments for ambulance rides—ranging from $289 to $481 in 2011—are far lower than commercial rates. Ambulance companies complain that Medicare rates do not meet the costs of running what are essentially mobile emergency rooms staffed by highly trained professionals.

In a recent study, the federal Health and Human Services Department's Office of the Inspector General noted that the Medicare ambulance services were "vulnerable to abuse and fraud," in part because there were lax standards on when an ambulance was needed and how the trip should be billed. The number of transports paid for by Medicare increased 69 percent between 2002 and 2011, while the number of Medicare patients increased only 7 percent during that period. In the last year, two ambulance companies have pleaded guilty or settled claims for overbilling Medicare.

Some will grant coverage [for ambulance service] if the destination was an emergency room, regardless of the patient's status, but others may require admittance to the hospital as evidence that the condition was serious. *"Insurers will generally cover if you had good reason to believe there was a serious threat to your life or health,"* said Susan Pisano, a spokeswoman for America's Health Insurance Plans, an industry group.

If you are a traditional ambulance provider, regardless of your type of governance, this article should scare you. The "value" of ambulance service is being questioned. On the other hand, if you have invested the time and resources to develop or begin developing an MIH program, you'll have data to demonstrate the value you bring to patients in the community and the payer. The value is generally not in tracking ambulance use and billing for transport (recall that emergency services are paid as a transportation benefit, not a healthcare benefit).

In the MIH environment, the demonstration of value is much different. You need to track and report data on patient outcomes, improvement in patient health status, patient experience of care, expenditure avoidance, and provider satisfaction. These measures need to relate to the value of the intervention that EMS provides in a healthcare environment. One of the only healthcare-related, clinical outcome measures that are traditionally reported is the cardiac arrest survival rate. Traditional EMS reporting often does not take a holistic approach to the various performance measures that should be included to determine the value of EMS to the healthcare delivery system.

Recording and Tracking Data

At MedStar, data recording in the tracking system starts with a key question: *What problem needs to be solved?* By asking yourself that question, it becomes clearer the kind of data you need to track. For example, if you're trying to reduce unnecessary EMS calls by implementing an EMS loyalty program, you would begin with some benchmark calculations on how much time, energy, effort, and money you're investing in treating patients or responding to patients who are frequent users of 9-1-1 for nonemergencies.

If you are developing a congestive heart failure (CHF) readmission reduction program, it would be important to know the current baseline metrics for CHF readmissions for aggregate and patient-specific calculations to determine whether your program is having a positive impact on patient outcomes. If you're working in partnership with one of your local hospitals to reduce the incidence of low-acuity patients visiting the ED, you need to know the impact those patients are having on the hospital before you begin tracking data. Developing baseline data is important for long-term measurement and will provide you with information to enable you to evaluate your program to demonstrate improvement in patient outcomes.

Another key point therefore needs to be addressed—what does success look like? Knowing the measures that will demonstrate the success and value of your MIH program will not only help you understand the data you should be tracking and reporting, but it will also help secure potential sustainable funding opportunities.

The conversation involved in developing a hospital partnership may be as follows:

MIH Agency: For a CHF readmission reduction program to demonstrate value to you, what percentage in reduction on readmissions for the enrolled patients would you like to see?

Hospital: For us, our current readmission rate is 24% for all CHF discharges. So, a reduction of at least 10% would be needed to make the program something we would financially support.

MIH Agency: For clarity, does that reduction of 10% mean that your readmission rate overall would fall 10%, meaning from 24% to 14%, or does it mean that the readmission rate would fall by 10%, from 24% to 21.6%?

Hospital: We mean for the rate to drop by 10% to 21.6% from 24%.

MIH Agency: To meet this goal, the agency would need to treat all CHF discharges to have an impact, because there may be patients who are readmitted who were not treated by the agency. Would it be more reasonable for the agency to have an impact on the readmission rate by enrolling patients into the MIH program and setting a goal of reducing the 30-day readmission rate of the enrolled patients by 50%? This would mean that if 30 patients were enrolled in the program, a reduction in readmission of 15 or more patients would be seen.

Hospital: Yes, that makes sense.

MIH Agency: If the agency is able to meet or exceed that outcome goal, would that demonstrate enough value for you to invest in the program long-term?

Hospital: Yes, definitely!

The focus of the discussion between the MIH agency and the hospital is on metrics and definitions. The conversation ensures that the MIH agency and the hospital have a clear understanding of the definition of success for the program. The discussion also allows for the opportunity to introduce the possibility of long-term funding for the successful program.

An EMS loyalty program can be developed using the same metrics and definitions of success. If your internal goal is to reduce the frequency of EMS or ED use in the enrolled population, you first need to determine the baseline measure of the current frequency of use in the target population. Then, apply your unit hour cost to the time committed on these calls. Next, a payer analysis evaluates whether any revenue is being generated from these calls. A payer analysis is a necessary component of the program to determine the potential loss of revenue from not transporting these patients.

The information you gather for this program will inform you that an EMS agency rarely demonstrates an internal cost savings by not responding to EMS loyalty program members unless you actually reduce costs. By eliminating transports, available unit hours will increase, but you will not see a cost savings unless you reduce unit hours. The same argument is true in the hospital environment. Reducing ED use for low-acuity patients may improve the efficiency at which the hospital is able to move patients through the ED, but unless the hospital is able to reduce staff, no direct cost savings to the hospital will be realized. This is a key point to consider when you are developing an EMS Loyalty program. It may be challenging to convince hospital partners to fund this program based on cost savings alone.

For the EMS provider, there is an argument to be made that not having to add unit hours to meet rising call volume is a cost savings, but the calculation to determine this type of cost savings is relatively complicated. At MedStar, the first fiscal year after the EMS loyalty program was implemented, four EMT positions were eliminated from the budget, and the four paramedic partner pairings for the EMTs were retained and used as staffing for MIH practitioner positions. As a specific example of how cost savings can be realized, for fiscal year 2009, MedStar scheduled 235,144 unit hours. A unit hour is one hour of a staffed ambulance, on-duty and available to respond to a call. In fiscal year 2010, MedStar reduced scheduled unit hours from the 235,144 in 2009, to 228,148, the equivalent of three on-duty ambulances. Reducing the EMT portion of budgeted unit hours saved MedStar approximately $200,000 in annual personnel costs.

Transparency in Outcome Reporting

At MedStar, the utilization data reported to the stakeholders is very specific. The development of a reporting process evolved over time and took months to perfect. The purity of data tracking and reporting assists with the ability to generate and publish data and helps with the replication of results.

Often, patients enrolled in EMS loyalty programs are transient, meaning they may move in and out of your community periodically. It is therefore important not to report outcomes that are derived from interventions that may not be specifically clinical or behavioral changes. For example, if one of the patients enrolled in MedStar's EMS loyalty program leaves the area and moves 1,000 miles away, it could be logically presumed that the reason for the decrease in 9-1-1 use in Fort Worth was because of the patient's geographic relocation rather than a change in behavior. A patient who has relocated to Key West may still be overusing the 9-1-1 system, but it is not possible to gather data from patients who are not available for follow up.

MedStar's data analysis reports only utilization data on patients who have been in the system for 2 years—1 year in MedStar's service prior to enrollment in the EMS loyalty program and 1 year in the service area after graduation from the program (**Table 7-2**). With this timeframe, MedStar could be confident that the change in patient utilization is the result of program participation, not geographic relocation.

Table 7-2 Utilization Analysis for One EMS Loyalty Program Patient

	911 Use					ED Visits				
Patient	**Pre-Enrollment**	**During Enrollment**	**% Change**	**Post Grad-uation**	**% Change**	**Pre-Enrollment**	**During Enrollment**	**% Change**	**Post Grad-uation**	**% Change**
Doe, John	110	60	−45.5%	20	−81.8%	121	71	−41.3%	28	−76.9%

To build on this data metric, MedStar applies the economic impact of this utilization change on costs. The following three terms are used to describe costs for healthcare services:

Cost: The *cost of delivering the service*, such as cost per unit hour, cost per transport, cost per ED hour staffed, and cost per patient seen

Charge: The amount *billed* for the services provided, such as the gross charges for the ambulance transport, ED visit, or admission. The charges have no real bearing on the amount *paid* for the service delivered. Billed charges are often referred to as "Monopoly" money—it is simply a number on paper.

Expenditure: The amount paid for the service provided.

Here's an example of how costs are calculated. One ambulance unit hour costs $138. This is a fully loaded cost, taking into account all fixed and variable costs to produce one unit hour such as personnel, equipment, supplies, fuel, and maintenance and overhead costs such as communications, billing, and administration. With a transport unit hour utilization of 0.355, each transport *costs* $388 ($138/0.355).

The gross average patient charge (APC) for a medically necessary ambulance transport in which advanced life support services are provided and Medicare pays the bill is $1,665. Of the $1,665 charge, Medicare allows a payment of $421. If the patient has met the deductible and coinsurance requirements, Medicare pays the $421. The balance cannot be billed to the patient, so the amount collected on the service and deposited into the bank is $421.

The application of the three types of costs is as follows:

Cost $388

Charge $1,665

Expenditure $421

For a payer analysis, and for most reporting, MedStar uses the *expenditure* savings because that is really the bottom line. With these metrics, a typical quarterly report for the EMS loyalty program is shown in **Table 7-3**.

Table 7-3 Sample Expenditure Savings Analysis

Expenditure Savings Analysis (1) EMS Loyalty Program			
Based on Medicare Rates			
Analysis Dates: **January 1, 2010–April 30, 2014**			
Number of Patients (2): **88**			
		CHP 9-1-1 Transports to ED	
Category	**Base**	**Avoided**	**Savings**
Ambulance Charge	$1,668	1629	$2,717,172
Ambulance Payment (3)	$427	1629	$695,583
ED Charges	$904	1629	$1,472,616
ED Payment (4)	$774	1629	$1,260,846
ED Bed Hours	6	1629	9,774
Total Charge Avoidance			**$4,189,788**
Total Payment Avoidance			**$1,956,429**
Per Patient Enrolled			**Community Health Program**
Charge Avoidance			**$47,611**
Payment Avoidance			**$22,232**

Notes:
1. Comparison based on use for 12 months prior to enrollment vs. 12 months after MIH graduation
2. Patients with data 12 months before and after graduation
3. Average Medicare payment received by MedStar
4. Base expenditures derived by AHRQ reports
Source: Data provided by John Peter Smith Health Network.

Obtaining Access to Patient Data

A question often asked during program discussions is how those involved in the program who are not the 9-1-1 provider can obtain access to utilization data on EMS loyalty patients. You have several options in this scenario. First, try to develop a relationship with the 9-1-1 provider that will enable them to share the data with you. There are also several other options to obtain the data. You could ask the patient. Patients will be willing to share their medical information with you if they have called 9-1-1. You could also ask the ED directors to share the information with you. The HIPAA privacy rule allows the sharing of health information for treatment, payment, and operations.[2]

Specifically, the rule states:

> The core health care activities of "Treatment," "Payment," and "Health Care Operations" [TPO clause] are defined in the Privacy Rule at 45 CFR 164.501.

"Treatment" generally means the provision, coordination, or management of health care and related services among health care providers or by a health care provider with a third party, consultation between health care providers regarding a patient, or the referral of a patient from one health care provider to another.

"Health care operations" are certain administrative, financial, legal, and quality improvement activities of a covered entity that are necessary to run its business and to support the core functions of treatment and payment.

These activities, which are limited to the activities listed in the definition of "health care operations" at 45 CFR 164.501, include:

Conducting quality assessment and improvement activities, population-based activities relating to improving health or reducing health care costs, and case management and care coordination.

On the basis of these definitions, it seems that the type of information exchanged among healthcare providers is permissible as part of the TPO clause of the HIPAA privacy rule.

An additional safeguard to help healthcare partners with HIPAA privacy issues is to have the patient sign a consent form with specific language authorizing the sharing of their information for care coordination. Patients in the MedStar programs sign the following statement as part of the enrollment process:

I hereby authorize the MedStar to release:

Any or all of my/the patient's medical information from and to the referring physicians, physician assistants, healthcare providers, including a public health nurse, or home health agency referral, insurance companies, and other third-party sponsors to facilitate healthcare, processing of claims, audit of payments for hospitalization and/or treatment, and to facilitate overall assessment of the CHP effectiveness. I understand that the information released may include records in these areas: HIV/AIDS, sexually transmitted disease, mental health treatment, and drug and alcohol abuse treatment; basic patient information regarding date and time of appointment(s) to family members (parents, spouses, adult children, guardians), and caregivers.

Clinical Record Keeping

In traditional EMS, patient charting is completed on an episode-based patient care report (ePCR). Once the field crew completes the chart and obtains the requisite signatures, the chart is uploaded to a billing system for processing. In most cases, retrieving previous patient records is not possible.

When you are caring for a patient in the MIH environment, having access to previous assessment records, vital sign trends, and educational instructions is paramount. Imagine that you are assessing a patient with CHF on a routine home visit who has been visited by two or three MIH

Being enrolled in the MedStar Mobile Health-care program was very beneficial. We were taught the importance of diet, medication, and living with congestive heart failure. The ability of the paramedic to make a call directly to the cardiologist or nephrologist when an issue comes up is wonderful. The doctors make adjustments as necessary while the paramedic is in the house. Having medications regulated without having to go back to the hospital has been nice. Being able to call this program instead of 9-1-1 when something isn't quite right is also a benefit. They come out all hours of the day or night to assist as needed. The paramedics are very personable and get to know their patients very well. We highly recommend this program.

Rick and Van Walker
MedStar MIH patients

practitioners over the past 3 weeks. The patient is complaining of slight dyspnea with some dependent edema and a 3-pillow orthopnea. To provide appropriate treatment, you should have access to the patient's previous assessment findings—weight, vital signs trending, and 12L ECG.

You may need this information for your assessment and to be able to share the history of treatment with the patient's primary care physician if necessary.

The essential difference between an ePCR and an electronic medical record (EMR) is that generally an ePCR will not be retrievable from the field, whereas an EMR would give the provider access to the patient's medical history and assessment findings. Having a robust EMR is a critical component in order to effectively operate an MIH program. At MedStar, an EMR was created using the Microsoft SharePoint program, because a viable electronic medical record for EMS has yet to be developed. The program was used to track vehicle maintenance requests, complaint tracking, and various other applications, which made it the first choice for developing a system for EMRs. There are many other software or web application platforms available that may meet the needs of your agency, and several EMS-based ePCR developers such as ESO Solutions, Image Trend, and Infor are actively working on the development of an EMR for EMS. An evaluation of the capabilities of the software will help you choose the right one for creating organizational intranets that are user friendly.

MedStar's SharePoint application is used to provide intranet portals, document and file management, collaboration, social networks, extranets, websites, enterprise search, and business intelligence. It also has system integration, process integration, and workflow automation capabilities. Data can be uploaded, downloaded, or even shared with hospitals or other care providers by either direct upload or by printing a PDF file and securely emailing it to requested recipients.

The following images are examples of the software screens used for the MIH programs.

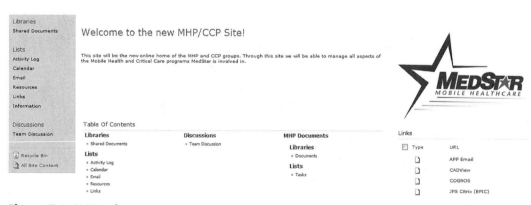

Figure 7-1 EMR welcome screen.

MedStar Mobile Healthcare, Fort Worth, TX.

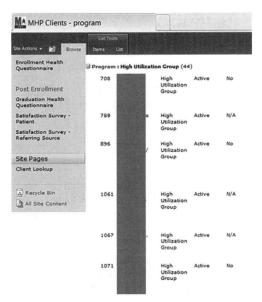

Figure 7-2 Electronic medical record patient summary screen. High utilization group refers to the EMS loyalty program members.

MedStar Mobile Healthcare, Fort Worth, TX.

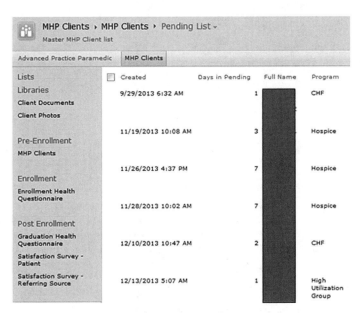

Figure 7-3 Electronic medical record pending patient enrollment screen.

MedStar Mobile Healthcare, Fort Worth, TX.

Data Tracking and Reporting for Hospice Revocation Avoidance

Data collection management can also be applied to hospice revocation. The clinical and economic challenges of patient disenrollment in hospice, whether voluntary or involuntary, have been discussed. To demonstrate value to the hospice agency (the payer of your MIH services in this case) you would need to know the percentage of voluntary disenrollments or revocations in the target enrollment-eligible patients. If these metrics improve, it means the patient's wishes are being met, and the hospice agency is saving money.

To collect and report the data necessary to prove value, the hospice agency should determine the cost of a voluntary disenrollment or revocation in terms of lost revenue and additional medical expenses. To assist you with ensuring the hospice agency is accounting for these expenses, sample data from the Centers for Medicare and Medicaid Services (CMS) regarding hospice are given in **Table 7-4**.

A study conducted by Mount Sinai Medical Center and published in the *Journal of Clinical Oncology*[3] analyzed 90,826 patients with cancer receiving hospice care. The study found that the cost of care for patients who disenrolled was more than five times the cost of not disenrolling and continuing to receive hospice care:[4]

> *Researchers at Mount Sinai School of Medicine have found that the costs of care for patients with cancer who disenrolled from hospice were nearly five times higher than for patients who remained with hospice. Patients who disenroll from hospice are far more likely to use emergency department care and be hospitalized.*

> *Nearly 11 percent of these patients disenrolled from hospice care and had significantly higher healthcare use and costs than those who remained in hospice until death.*

Table 7-4 CMS Hospice Categories

Category	Description	Base Payment Rate
Routine home care	Home care provided on a typical day	$151 per day
Continuous home care	Home care provided during periods of patient crisis	$36.73 per hour
Inpatient respite care	Inpatient care for a short period to provide respite for primary caregiver	$156 per day
General inpatient care	Inpatient care to treat symptoms that cannot be managed in another setting	$672 per day

Note: FY (fiscal year). Payment for continuous home care (CHC) is an hourly rate for care delivered during periods of crisis if care is provided in the home for 8 or more hours within a 24-hour period beginning at midnight. A nurse must deliver more than half of the hours of this care to qualify for CHC-level payment. The minimum daily payment rate at the CHC level is $294 per day (8 hours at $36.73 per hour); maximum daily payment at the CHC level is $881 per day (24 hours at $36.73 per hour).

Reproduced from CMS Manual System Pub 100-04 Medicare Claims Processing, Transmittal 22260, Update to Hospice Payment Rates, Hospice Cap, Hospice Wage Index, and Hospice prices for FY 2012. July 29, 2011.

Patients with cancer who disenrolled from hospice were more likely to be hospitalized (39.8% vs. 1.6%; P < .001), more likely to be admitted to the emergency department (33.9% vs. 3.1%; P < .001) or intensive care unit (5.7% vs. 0.1%; P < .001), and more likely to die in the hospital (9.6% vs. 0.2%; P < .001).

Patients who disenrolled from hospice died a median of 24 days following disenrollment, suggesting that the reason for hospice disenrollment was not improved health. In multivariable analyses, hospice disenrollees incurred higher per-day Medicare expenditures than patients who remained with hospice until death (higher per-day expenditures of $124; P < .001).

If you apply these metrics to the hospice point of view, the lost revenue per disenrolled hospice patient is $3,600 (24 days × $151/day). Then, if you apply the cost to the hospice agency of one ambulance trip, plus the cost of an ED visit and a day or two of inpatient status prior to disenrollment, that expense could easily be another $4,000–$6,000 or more. This calculation brings the total potential loss to the hospice agency to $7,000–$10,000.

An analysis of the patients enrolled in MedStar's Hospice Revocation Avoidance program is given in **Table 7-5**.

Note the 11% revocation rate in the population in the table. The patients referred into this program, based on the hospice agency's risk assessment, are at high risk for voluntary disenrollment, or revocation. The 11% revocation rate in these patients is viewed as a significant improvement for the hospice agency.

Table 7-5 Hospice Program Summary Data

Hospice Program Summary		
As of April 30, 2014		
	No.	**%**
Referrals	154	
Enrolled	129	
Deceased	81	62.8%
Active	33	25.6%
Improved	2	1.6%
Revoked	**13**	**10.1%**
Activity		
9-1-1 calls	11	
9-1-1 transports	5	
ED visits	3	
Direct Admits	2	

The data collection and analysis for this MIH program involve more than simply looking at ambulance response or transport data.

Patient and Provider Satisfaction—The Stakeholder Experience

In June 2012, MedStar presented the MIH programs and their outcomes to a select group of researches and biostatisticians from the Agency for Healthcare Research and Quality (AHRQ). AHRQ is a research and policy arm of Health and Human Services (HHS); they rate innovations based on outcome measures. After a data-laden presentation to a group of researchers, the first question from the audience was "What do the patients think about the programs?"—an excellent question that had no immediate answer. As a result of this presentation and discussion, a patient experience survey was developed. MedStar not only included the experience of the patient, but the experience of the person making the referral also. **Table 7-6** provides recent examples of the patient experience evaluations.

With a health status survey tool, MedStar was able to report data on the patient's change in health status.

Table 7-6 Patient Satisfaction Analysis for MedStar MIH Program

As of: 7/31/2013	CHP	CHF	NTSP
Sample Size	**70**	**75**	**61**
MHP listened to your concerns	4.86	4.84	5.00
MHP took time to answer your questions	5.00	4.88	4.95
Overall amount of time spent with you	5.00	4.72	4.95
MHP explanations were easy to understand	4.86	4.84	4.90
MHP gave written instructions for managing your illness	4.86	4.76	5.00
Completeness of examinations	5.00	4.80	4.95
MHP gave advice to manage your illness	5.00	4.76	4.57
Quality of medical care	5.00	4.88	5.00
Level of compassion	5.00	4.96	5.00
Overall Satisfaction	**4.86**	**4.92**	**5.00**

Notes: Scale is from 1–5, with 5 representing most satisfied. CHP indicates community health program; CHF, congestive heart failure program; NTSP, North Texas Specialty Physician's Observational Admission Avoidance program.

Table 7-7 Health Status Indicator Changes—MedStar MIH Programs

Patient Self-Assessment of Health Status (1) As of: 7/31/2013	CHP			CHF			NTSP		
	Pre	Post	Change	Pre	Post	Change	Pre	Post	Change
Sample Size	**12**	**10**		**26**	**26**		**8**	**18**	
Mobility (2)	2.417	2.300	−4.8%	2.346	2.615	11.5%	2.750	2.611	−5.1%
Self-Care (2)	2.583	2.500	−3.2%	2.423	2.654	9.5%	2.750	2.667	−3.0%
Perform Usual Activities (2)	2.333	2.300	−1.4%	2.269	2.500	10.2%	2.750	2.556	−7.1%
Pain and Discomfort (2)	1.667	2.400	44.0%	2.154	2.423	12.5%	2.750	2.444	−11.1%
Axiety/Depression (2)	1.667	2.000	20.0%	2.154	2.346	8.9%	2.750	2.722	−1.0%
Overall Health Status (3)	**3.3**	**6.6**	**98.0%**	**5.4**	**7.1**	**32.1%**	**6.8**	**6.8**	**0.4%**

Notes:

1. Average scores of preenrollment and postenrollment data from EuroQol EQ-5D-3L Assessment Questionnaire
2. Score 1–3, with 3 most favorable
3. Score 1–10, with 10 most favorable

Data Tracking and Reporting for 9-1-1 Nurse Triage

For the 9-1-1 Nurse Triage program, MedStar built a similar metric for measuring the calls referred to the nurse, the calls that received a disposition other than an ambulance to the emergency department, and the patient's satisfaction with the care received. Referring to the costs, charges, and expenditures for the program, MedStar's data revealed the results given in **Tables 7-8** and **7-9** and **Figure 7-5**.

Take special note of the patient satisfaction scores for the patients who received a disposition other than an ambulance to the emergency department. One might presume that patients who called 9-1-1 and did not receive an ambulance response would be less than satisfied with that outcome. MedStar's data revealed the opposite.

Changing Metrics

Creating new metrics for measuring performance is not unique to EMS or MIH. In a recent article published in *Hospitals and Health Networks*, OhioHealth President and CEO David Blom explained how the metrics in the hospital world is changing[5]:

> The success factors are the same today as they were in the past, but the metrics are changing. For instance, market share can't be defined by volume anymore, but rather by attributed lives. Process measures for quality? Hardly; try clinical integration. Profitability will be defined by managing risk, not by high volumes. Physician relations? How about economic integration. And, importantly, the focus on access has shifted from inpatient to ambulatory.

By placing a checkmark in one box in each group below, please indicate which statements best describe your own health state today.

Mobility

I have no problems in walking about ☐

I have some problems in walking about ☐

I am confined to bed ☐

Self-Care

I have no problems with self-care ☐

I have some problems washing or dressing myself ☐

I am unable to wash or dress myself ☐

Usual Activities (*e.g. work, study, housework, family or leisure activities*)

I have no problems with performing my usual activities ☐

I have some problems with performing my usual activities ☐

I am unable to perform my usual activities ☐

Pain/Discomfort

I have no pain or discomfort ☐

I have moderate pain or discomfort ☐

I have extreme pain or discomfort ☐

Anxiety/Depression

I am not anxious or depressed ☐

I am moderately anxious or depressed ☐

I am extremely anxious or depressed ☐

Figure 7-4 Health status survey. (*Continues*)

To help people say how good or bad a health state is, we have drawn a scale (rather like a thermometer) on which the best state you can imagine is marked 100 and the worst state you can imagine is marked 0.

We would like you to indicate on this scale how good or bad your own health is today, in your opinion. Please do this by drawing a line from the box below to whichever point on the scale indicates how good or bad your health state is today.

Best
Imaginable
Health State

100

90

80

70

60

50

40

30

20

10

0

Worst
Imaginable
Health State

**Your Own
Health State
Today**

Figure 7-4 Health status survey. (*Continued*)

Oemar M, Oppe M,. EQ-5D-3L User Guide: Basic information on how to use the EQ-5D-3L instrument. http://www.euroqol.org/fileadmin/user_upload/Documenten/PDF/Folders_Flyers/EQ-5D-3L_UserGuide_2013_v5.0_October_2013.pdf

Table 7-8 MedStar 9-1-1 Nurse Triage Economic Analysis

Expenditure Savings Analysis (1) 9-1-1 Nurse Triage Program			

Based on Medicare Rates

Analysis Dates: **June 1, 2012–May 31, 2014**

Number of Calls Referred: **1,620**

% of Calls Alternatively Disposed: **40.6%**

Category	Base	9-1-1 Transports to ED Avoided	Savings
Ambulance Charge	$1,668	658	$1,097,544
Ambulance Payment (2)	$427	658	$280,966
ED Charges	$904	658	$594,832
ED Payment (3)	$774	658	$509,292
ED Bed Hours	6	658	3,948
Total Charge Avoidance			**$1,692,376**
Total Payment Avoidance			**$790,258**
Per Patient Enrolled			**Nurse Triage Program**
Charge Avoidance			**$2,572**
Payment Avoidance			**$1,201**

Notes:

1. Comparison based on use for 12 months prior to enrollment vs. 12 months after MIH graduation.

2. Average Medicare payment received by MedStar.

3. Base expenditures derived from AHRQ reports.

Data from: John Peter Smith Health Network

Table 7-9 MedStar 9-1-1 Nurse Patient Satisfaction Scores

Condition Got Better	Call Handled Different? = No	Talking to Nurse Helped
85.8%	76.8%	89.6%

A Word About Patient Safety

MIH programs are very new. Although the early data are exceptionally encouraging, the focus on patient safety has to be part of the metrics that are purposefully designed and reported on. Seeing patients in a nonemergency, prescheduled home visit and recommending methods for more effectively managing their healthcare comes with some risk. Data that track patient safety are essential. Some patient safety measures that should be tracked and reported are listed in the following sections.

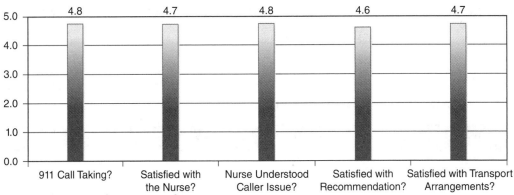

Figure 7-5 Graph of patient satisfaction scores.
Note: Scale is from 1–5, with 5 representing most satisfied.
Data from: MedStar Mobile Healthcare.

Nurse Triage

Nurse triage data consist of the following measures:

- Number and percentage of patients who died within 24 hours from a cause related to the reason for the ECNS contact call

- Number and percentage of patients who re-call 9-1-1 and get an ambulance response within 24 hours for a related complaint

- Number and percentage of patients who were triaged as low acuity and went to ED on their own and were admitted to a critical care unit

- Number and percentage of patients who follow recommendations and report a worsening condition on a 24-hour call-back to check on patient status

High-Utilizer Patients

High-utilizer data consist of the following measures:

- Number and percentage of patients who are *not* identified by the community paramedic during a home visit to be at risk for acute care admission and are subsequently admitted to a critical care unit or die within 48 hours

- Number and percentage of protocol deviations without specific medical direction supporting the deviation

- Number and percentage of patients referred to community partners for reconciliation of immediate social/environmental hazards and risks

Specific Diseases (such as CHF/Diabetes/Observation Admittance Avoidance)

- Number and percentage of protocol deviations without specific medical direction supporting the deviation

- Number and percentage of prescribed drug interaction/overprescription hazards discovered by community paramedics and referred to PCMH for reconciliation

Pearls of WISDOM

1. Don't assume value! Your stakeholders and payers will have a different view of value than you will. Be sure to ask them key questions to determine their view of value, and track and report data that matters to your them. Also ask them how they would like the data presented.

2. Be totally clear about the way you are reporting the data. For example, there are a few different ways to report a change in ED utilization, if that is one of your programs. You could measure the frequency of change from one period to the next, the absolute change for patients enrolled in the program. You could even measure the change in overall ED utilization per capita in your service area.

3. Know the difference between a percentage change and a rate of change measure. For example, if a hospice agency reports a revocation rate of 20% on April 1, and on September 1 their revocation rate is 15%, you could easily say the revocation rate dropped 5% (20 − 15 = 5), which would be accurate. However, it could also be reported that the revocation rate dropped *by* 25% and be accurate as well. The *rate* of change is measured by subtracting the new value from the old value and dividing it by the old value ([15 − 20]/20 in our example).

Are You READY?

- Read the Health Resources and Services Administration's Community Paramedic Evaluation Tool at: http://www.hrsa.gov/ruralhealth/pdf/paramedicevaltool.pdf

- Conduct a meeting with various external stakeholders to discuss relevant metrics they would consider useful in measuring the outcome performance of an MIH program.

- Read the Agency for Healthcare Research and Quality (AHRQ) report called *Data-Driven System Helps Emergency Medical Services Identify Frequent Callers and Connect Them to Community Services, Reducing Transports and Costs* at: http://www.innovations.ahrq.gov/content.aspx?xml:id=4073

- Read the *National Consensus Conference on Community Paramedicine: Summary of an Expert Meeting* document at: http://depts.washington.edu/uwrhrc/uploads/CP_Report.pdf

Summary

The data used, tracked, and reported in an MIH program are significantly different than data collection in a traditional EMS program. The gathering of data and reporting should be based on the stakeholder's definition of success and done in a way that is meaningful to the stakeholder. Be sure you have processes in place that can accurately and succinctly report meaningful data, and measure, track, and report patient satisfaction scores.

References

1. Rosenthal E. Think the E.R. is expensive? Look at how much it costs to get there. *NY Times* Health section. Available at: http://www.nytimes.com/2013/12/05/health/think-the-er-was-expensive-look-at-the-ambulance-bill.html?hp&_r=1&. Accessed June 25, 2014.

2. US Department of Health and Human Services. Uses and disclosures for treatment, payment, and healthcare. Available at: http://www.hhs.gov/ocr/privacy/hipaa/understanding/coveredentities /usesanddisclosuresfortpo.html. Accessed June 25, 2014.

3. Carlson MDA, Herrin J, Du Q, et al. Impact of hospice disenrollment on healthcare use and Medicare expenditures for patients with cancer [abstract]. *Am J Clin Oncol.* Available at: http://jco .ascopubs.org/content/early/2010/08/23/JCO.2009.26.1818.abstract. Accessed June 25, 2014.

4. Mount Sinai Hospital. Increased costs, hospitalizations seen in people with cancer who leave hospice early [press release]. Available at: http://www.mountsinai.org/about-us/newsroom/press-releases/ increased-costs-hospitalizations-seen-in-people-with-cancer-who-leave-hospice-care-early. Accessed June 25, 2014.

5. Weinstock M. Making the pivot. *Hospitals and Health Networks.* Available at: http://www.hhnmag .com/display/HHN-news-article.dhtml?dcrPath=/templatedata/HF_Common/NewsArticle/data/HHN/ Magazine/2014/Jun/healthmatters-value-based-transformation-ACO. Accessed June 25, 2014.

8

Funding Models for Mobile Integrated Healthcare

The statement below is a common comment from many agencies that have contacted MedStar about how to start an MIH program in their community:

> *It all comes down to money. We've been getting paid for transport for 30 years. I cannot convince my chief to invest in any of this MIH stuff without funding, and we're not going to get it from the city. What funding is available for MIH programs?*

City Fire Department EMS Chief

To enter into a discussion of funding an MIH program, it's important to consider the history of EMS as a profession and its role in the healthcare system. A fundamental change to healthcare system finance is occurring under the new accountable care environment created by the Affordable Care Act. As discussed in earlier chapters, a foundational shift is occurring from a traditional fee-for-service delivery model to payment mechanisms based on patient outcomes and meeting the IHI Triple Aim measures.

Ambulance *transport* has been a qualified patient benefit through the Centers for Medicare and Medicaid Services (CMS) as a "supplier" of medical services—transportation—not a "provider" of medical services, such as an outpatient clinic or home health agency. To survive in the new healthcare environment, EMS needs to become a provider of healthcare services.

MIH Funding Sources

The funding sources for MIH programs can be classified into the components given in **Table 8-1**.

Table 8-1 Sources of Funding for an MIH Program

Seed Funding	Sustainable Revenue
Grant	Fee for service
Community foundations	Patient contact
Hospital foundations	Referral
Center for Medicare and Medicaid Services Innovation	Outcome
	Shared savings

(Continues)

Table 8-1 Sources of Funding for an MIH Program (*Continued*)

Seed Funding	Sustainable Revenue
Cost Avoidance	Subscription based
Internally generated savings	Individual
	Corporate
Sponsorship(s)	Sponsorship(s)
Hospitals	Hospitals
Healthcare providers	Healthcare providers
Healthcare payers	Healthcare payers

Follow the Money

When you change how healthcare services are delivered to meet the IHI Triple Aim, financial benefits will be seen throughout the healthcare industry. Some gains will be short term, and others will be long term. For example, for a patient insured with UnitedHealthcare, preventing an unnecessary ambulance trip to the ED and navigating that patient to an appointment with a primary care physician *immediately* creates financial benefits for the payer through a reduced expenditure for that episode of care.

A reduction in the readmission rate will be a financial benefit for a hospital currently receiving a financial penalty for a high readmission rate, but it may take 2–3 years for the hospital to see that benefit because of the way the readmission rates are measured over time. Furthermore, you could reduce the readmission rate for *all* the patients referred into your CHF readmission prevention program, but due to other factors in the hospital, their overall readmission rate did not decrease. In determining the correct source for potential funding of your MIH program, follow the money! You should be talking about funding with the sources that are benefiting financially from the changes in the way you provide healthcare.

Seed or Start-up Funding

For agencies starting MIH programs, initial seed funding is often the greatest challenge. The good news is that, unlike in 2009 when MedStar started its programs, MIH is no longer considered an unknown risk. You can build on the successes of programs in Fort Worth, Texas; Wake County, North Carolina; Eagle County, Colorado; and western Pennsylvania to help make your financial argument supporting MIH programs. Data from these programs offer the answer to the inevitable question from the funder "What's in it for me?" Use outcome data from these programs to help make your case.

Choosing Your First Program

It is vital to choose a program based on local community needs. Knowing what's needed in the community will help with finding start-up funding because there may be partnering organizations willing to fund the initial program. For example, if your local hospital is looking for a partnership to reduce readmissions for patients with heart failure, they may be willing to invest in an MIH program to meet that goal. If the hospital is unable or unwilling to provide the funding for the start-up, they may have a foundation that is able to grant the funding to you for the start-up venture. Similarly, if one of the critical needs determined in your community is improving healthcare for the homeless, and the stated mission of a local community foundation is to help the homeless, you may find the foundation willing to fund a program you provide to bring healthcare to the homeless in a setting that improves their overall health status. This is why choosing the program is vital to finding the right funding source.

Cost Avoidance

Providing healthcare services is expensive, and attempts to gain cost efficiency are admirable. However, reducing costs for services that typically have a high fixed overhead or significant cost of readiness components can be challenging. A reduction in the number of services provided to a specific patient does not necessarily translate to a reduction in the total cost of providing those services for the agency. For example, if your MIH program addresses the needs of patients in an EMS loyalty program, unless you lower the rate of utilization enough to be able to reduce the number of ambulances deployed on the street, you will not realize a cost savings.

Sample Cost Avoidance Case Study

A sample case involves Jane Smith, an EMS loyalty patient who has called 9-1-1 for transport to a local ED an average of 10 times a month over the past 6 months. Most would agree this pattern fits the profile of an EMS loyalty patient. In your EMS system, you respond to 50,000 calls annually with a fleet of 22 ambulances staffed 24/7. Jane Smith is 40 years old, homeless, and became addicted to narcotic pain killers after a back injury 2 years ago. She also has a history of alcohol abuse, hypertension, asthma, and diabetes. You implement an MIH EMS loyalty patient program, and Jane Smith is your first patient.

After your first few proactive visits at her bridge overpass at 1st and Main, you begin to more fully understand her needs. As a result, you arrange the following for her well-being:

- Thirty days of temporary shelter at a women's shelter in your city

- Enrollment into the county-funded behavioral health system for treatment of her substance abuse

- Enrollment into the county-funded indigent care program, allowing her access to the 12 clinics in the county operated for indigent patients that she can now use as her patient-centered medical home

- Bus passes to allow her to go back and forth from her behavioral health clinic visits as often as she needs to, as well as to the pharmacy or other healthcare resources

- A nonemergency number to call you in case she needs any medical assessment or care—an alternative to calling 9-1-1.

As a result of this coordinated care that better meets her medical needs, Jane Smith reduces her 9-1-1 and ED use from 10 visits a month to 2 visits. With these data, you are able to create a cost savings analysis (**Table 8-2**).

Table 8-2 Cost Savings Analysis for Jane Smith

MIH 9-1-1 Transports to ED			
Category	**Base**	**Avoided**	**Savings**
Ambulance Cost	$750	8	$6,000
ED Cost	$500	8	$4,000
Total Savings			$10,000

With this incredible cost savings success, you hold a breakfast meeting with the EMS chief and the hospital administrator to explain the cost savings achieved with only one patient. After your presentation, however, the EMS chief tells you that you have not saved the agency any money. He says "Although you reduced the number of responses in the system by 8 calls, all 22 ambulances were still staffed for the month. In fact, you reduced the potential for billing for those 8 calls." You explain that the patient does not have a payer source; consequently, her trips do not generate revenue for the agency. The EMS chief tells you that the agency recently started receiving payments from the state government for uncompensated care based on the cost of delivering service that does not receive payment.

The hospital administrator also tells you that you have not saved the hospital any money. She says "You reduced the number of ED visits in the hospital by 8 for the month, but 4,000 patients a month are treated in the ED. The staffing and resources needed to be maintained for the other 3,992 visits." You explain, as you did with the EMS chief, that the patient does not have a payer source and therefore her ED visits don't generate revenue. As a result, you conclude that the hospital reduces their bad debt expense. The hospital administrator tells you that bad debt is simply an entry on an income statement to show the accounts they were unable to collect based on the total gross revenue (billed) services. In this case, the reduction in bad debt only occurs because there was a decrease in the billable services by 8 ED visits—a zero sum game.

The EMS chief and hospital administrator reinforce the rationale that cost savings only occur when you are able to reduce dollars spent on delivering care. If the EMS chief were able to reduce the number of staffed ambulance hours, thereby reducing unit hour costs, there is a *realized* cost savings. Similarly, for the hospital administrator, ED staff could not be reduced by eliminating 8 of 4,000 ED visits. Therefore, there is no *realized* cost savings.

A *cost avoidance* funding model for the EMS agency would have to reduce ambulance staffing at an amount equal to the cost of the MIH program. If your program costs $250,000 annually and the cost of one ambulance unit hour in your system is $135, you'd need to reduce ambulance staffing by nearly 2,000 hours annually—the equivalent of one ambulance Monday through Friday, from 9 am to 5 pm.

Sponsorship Funding and Sustainable Revenue

Sponsorship funding for an MIH program means that you find a funding partner who is willing to work with you on an initial demonstration project. Generally, this partner is a payer who will benefit in the long term from a successful MIH program.

An example of this type of funding is MedStar's 9-1-1 Nurse Triage program. MedStar knew that similar programs initiated in other cities were not successful partly because navigation of patients was difficult without an available network of resources. MedStar took a different approach and sought sponsorship from the hospital systems for the initial year. The sponsorship included funding the cost of the first triage nurse, which was approximately $90,000. MedStar covered the cost of the hardware, software, and other related costs, totaling another $100,000.

There were two main reasons for seeking the sponsorship. First, MedStar believed that if the hospitals had a vested financial interest in the program's success, they would help with any gateway issues related to access to clinics, primary care physician offices, or other alternative healthcare resources. Second, MedStar wanted to test the willingness of hospitals to make investments into the reform of the emergency care delivery system.

The hospitals were willing to sponsor the program using a balanced funding model (each of the four hospital systems paying 25% of the cost of the nurse) for the first year as a demonstration project. Hospitals did not fund the project because they believed the system would save them direct costs. They funded the project to find a solution for the penalties imposed on hospitals for low patient satisfaction ratings. Low-acuity patients who call 9-1-1 are typically delivered by ambulance to triage and generally are placed in a waiting room where they could wait 6–8 hours for treatment. When patients are finally evaluated, they usually need to be referred to another source of care (such as a dentist for a toothache or a pain management specialist for pain medication).

Ten percent of patients admitted to the ED receive a patient satisfaction questionnaire in the mail a few days after their visit. The patient ratings are generally poor because of the long waiting time and because the ED was unable to provide the patient with the treatment needed. If patients are triaged to a more appropriate source of care rather than the ED, the patient satisfaction survey results will most likely improve. Navigating low-acuity patients to the correct resources for their care prevents them from ever receiving an HCAPHS survey and improves their patient experience. By reducing the number of low-acuity patients in the ED waiting room, the waiting time for other patients may also be reduced, potentially improving their satisfaction rating of the experience.

Knowing the value of your proposition for your potential customers will help you make a case for either seed money or sustainable funding. The hospitals in the MedStar community have renewed their support for the 9-1-1 nurse triage program by funding it beyond the first year demonstration project.

This is just one example of acquiring seed money for start-up. Insurance companies and other healthcare providers such as hospice agencies, home health agencies, or skilled nursing facilities may be equally interested in funding the programs that financially help them. Several models for sustainable funding are available, again, depending on finding the payer or provider who is benefiting from the MIH program. Some examples from MedStar's experience follow which could apply to your community.

Patient Contact Fees

MedStar has fee-for-service contracts with two payers. One hospital pays a per-patient contact fee to help manage EMS loyalty patients and reduce unnecessary ED visits. A case manager in the hospital identifies a patient who will benefit from the EMS loyalty program, discusses the program and enrollment with the patient, and if the patient agrees to enroll, sends the referral forms to MedStar to make contact with the patient. The hospital pays a fee for each patient visit. If one patient has 10 visits for the month, the hospital pays the fee for 10 patient visits.

Another patient contact fee contract is with a home health agency. The home health agency contacts MedStar as a backup to the agency's on-call home health nurse on nights and weekends. It is more cost effective for the agency to have an MIH practitioner do an episodic home visit than to pay a home health nurse overtime for making the visit. Most of the time, the episodic visit request is for a situation that an MIH practitioner can assess and then discuss with the home health nurse on-call to determine the most appropriate patient care.

Visionary leaders have worked to pass legislation that allows Medicaid to pay for MIH services. These arrangements are largely on a fee for service/patient contact model as long as certain training, certification, and other parameters are met. Medicare does not currently pay for ambulance response without transport for medical conditions other than deceased patients on scene. However, they *do* have a HCPCS code assigned to this delivery model (*A0998 – Ambulance response and treatment, no transport*) in the event it becomes funded in the future, and to allow billing a patient for the service if it is denied by Medicare.[1] As with any service EMS provides, it is permissible to bill the patient. However, direct patient billing for services may dramatically change the referral process to avoid running afoul of self-referral and kickback statutes. The federal Anti-Kickback Statute (42 USC § 1320a-7b(b)) prohibits offering, paying, soliciting, or receiving anything of value to induce or reward referrals or generate federal healthcare program business. The law is intended to address the concern that financial incentives have a tendency to corrupt the medical decision making of those providing care. As such, the government wants to ensure that medical decisions are made in the best interests of patients.[2] If a provider solicits a patient to enroll in a healthcare services program for which the

VOICES OF EXPERIENCE

VITAS Innovative Hospice-Fort Worth is so proud to work with MedStar and their community health program. Over the past 2 years MedStar and their mobile health paramedics have proven to be a great support for and partner to VITAS hospice staff as we endeavor to care for the community's most medically complex patients in their own home. The MedStar/VITAS community collaboration has enabled VITAS-Fort Worth to keep our revocation rates well below the national average and our family satisfaction high. We are grateful for our collaboration with MedStar.

Monica Cushion
Director of Market Development
VITAS Healthcare
Fort Worth, Texas

provider intends to receive payment for, that could be easily perceived as a kickback. In the MIH scenario, if you use your own ambulance response records (a billable service) to identify a patient you'd like to enroll in a EMS loyalty program (another billable service) then it's possible you could be found in violation of the anti-kickback statutes.

Many EMS agencies, including MedStar, bill the patient for a treatment-no transport given certain conditions. If a response is made to a first- or second-party call (a call in which the patient or immediate family member with the patient) calls 9-1-1 with an advanced assessment and/or some from treatment, the patient is billed for the on-scene treatment. Treatment of a hypoglycemic diabetic patient is a good example. On arrival, the patient receives a full assessment, and it is determined the medically appropriate course of treatment is administration of IV dextrose. The patient becomes alert and oriented and then refuses transport. The patient is billed $126.50 for the response, assessment, and treatment. When a third-party payer is billed (private insurance), the collection rate is 53%. More and more insurance companies are willing to pay the fee to avoid downstream costs, including the $1,000 ambulance fee.

A cautionary note for billing for these services is that in some cases the agency may be seeking to have the patient enrolled in the MIH program, such as the internal EMS loyalty program referral. Make sure that it does not appear that you are self-referring patients into a program for which they will be billed by you. Similarly, if you are billing privately for home visits for patients referred to you by other healthcare providers, such as hospitals, your service delivery model may be viewed as competitive.

Referral Fees

MedStar has two referral fee contracts, one with a hospital and one with a payer (ACO). For the hospital contract, under the previously described 1115 waiver project made possible through the ACA, a large county hospital system pays MedStar a per-patient enrolled fee for the patients listed in **Table 8-3**.

Table 8-3 Patients Enrolled in MIH Program for a Fee

Type	Goal
EMS loyalty program group	Reduce preventable ED visits
CHF	Reduce preventable readmissions
Observational admit	Reduce observational admissions
9-1-1 nurse triage	Reduce unnecessary ED visits

For each patient enrolled in an MIH program, the hospital pays a fee. For example, the hospital pays $800 for a CHF patient enrolled in the MedStar program, regardless of the number of times the patient is seen by an MIH practitioner. Additionally, if MedStar meets specific program objectives that are mutually agreed upon, a bonus payment may be awarded at the end of the year.

The second referral fee contract is with the payer. A contract with the payer (formerly part of an ACO) allows them to refer an at-risk patient who has been released from the ED for a 23-hour observation to an MIH program.

Rather than patients being held in the ED overnight for observation, they are referred to MedStar to have an MIH practitioner visit the patient's home once or twice between discharge and their appointment with a follow-up provider (primary care physician or specialist). A per-referral fee is paid by the payer for this service.

Outcome-Based Payments

Outcome-based payments are the future of MIH services. The entire healthcare industry is moving toward outcome-based payments. MedStar has one outcome-based contract and is transitioning two of the previously discussed contracts to this model. This financial model closely follows the concept of shared savings, which are discussed in more detail later.

Hospice service fits well into this payment model. The hospice agency identifies a patient or patient family believed to be at high risk for voluntary hospice disenrollment or revocation. The MIH program is described to them to gauge their interest in the additional support service at no cost to them. If the patient and family agree, the patient is referred to MedStar for enrollment in the hospice disenrollment avoidance program.

If an enrolled hospice patient dies without a voluntary disenrollment or revocation, MedStar receives a payment. If the patient disenrolls or hospice status is revoked, MedStar does not get paid. Payment is based on patient outcome, and, in most cases, MIH practitioners have minimal interaction with the patient. Practitioners are available mainly as an additional safety net if the family members become scared or panic. The financial model is based on a shared saving concept. If the patient stays in service with hospice without excessive healthcare services expenses, the hospice agency has a significant financial gain that will be shared with the MIH agency.

Shared Savings Model

The shared savings model works well for programs in which a stakeholder realizes a cost savings. The observation admission avoidance program is a logical fit for a shared savings model. If the payer, in this case, the ACO, avoids having to pay for the observation admission because they have referred the patient into your MIH program, they have an expenditure savings (for MedStar locally, it's about $8,000 for the payer). If the patient is not readmitted to the ED and transitions safely to a follow-up appointment, the payer shares a percentage of their savings. The 80/20 rule has been used by CMS for other shared savings programs; therefore, MedStar has proposed that the payer retain 80% of the savings and pay the MIH provider 20% of the savings.

Table 8-4 Expenditure Savings Analysis

Observation Admission Avoidance Program **Analysis Dates: August 1, 2012, to April 30, 2014** **Observation Admits Avoided**					
Category	**Base**	**Avoided**	**Gross Savings**	**Enrollment Fees**	**Net Savings**
Average Observation Admit Expense	$8,046	87	$700,002	$17,400	**$682,602**
ED Bed Hours	23	87			**2,001**
Per patient enrolled					**Observation Admit**
Payment avoidance					$7,846

Using the example in **Table 8-4**, you could generate $130,000 annually for your program if you enrolled 5–10 patients a month into the observation admission avoidance program.

Individual Subscriptions

Many EMS agencies are familiar with the concept of a membership, or subscription program. A subscription is typically an annual fee paid to the provider in which the subscriber (and perhaps his or her immediate family members sharing the same residence) has co-insurance and deductibles waived for a nominal fee. The program at MedStar has been active for 25 years and currently has more than 9,000 members. Imagine that you take those memberships to a new level to include the option for MIH. As a MedStar member, not only do you have the financial benefit as mentioned previously, but you are provided a 24/7 nonemergency access number to request an MIH provider home visit for a low-acuity assessment and a special number to access the triage nurse, from 8 am to 8 pm, 7 days a week. If a member is willing to pay, for example, $20 annually, then $20 times 8,000 members is a financial benefit of $160,000 annually. Your agency would need to manage the resource properly, based on the utilization by possibly setting limits of four home visits a year.

Another subscription opportunity can be offered for the care of newborns. The MedStar new arrivals program subscription will enable an MIH practitioner to visit the house, perform a child safety review of the home, help identify any issues that the parents may want to address, and present an infant/child CPR class for the parents and anyone else they want to invite. The subscription also provides a nonemergency access number for a nurse between 8 am and 8 pm, 7 days a week, to ask questions. The subscription also provides four home visits 24/7 throughout the year by an MIH practitioner for any child healthcare. How much would that be worth to parents—$100, $500? The new arrivals program provides additional peace of mind for the parents and access to immediate nonemergency care for the child. The program can be an additional revenue stream for your agency.

Another important opportunity for a subscription program lies at the opposite end of the life spectrum. For example, many elderly people have some medical issues but are reasonably healthy and active. They are not candidates for an assisted living center, but their children worry about them. And to complicate the situation, they live in another state, and the children cannot see them as often as they would like. A MedStar safe transitions subscription can provide key assistance for them. Upon enrollment, an MIH practitioner will visit the home and perform a safety assessment, focusing on fall hazards. The subscribers would also be provided hands-only CPR training and access to a nonemergency number for a nurse between 8 am and 8 pm, 7 days a week, to ask questions and to request up to four home visits 24/7 throughout the year by an MIH practitioner. A safe transitions program can provide revenue for your agency and help families with aging loved ones receive the care they need.

Corporate Subscriptions

This same concept for subscriptions can be applied to employers to offer as an employee benefit. The employer also benefits from this arrangement by potentially reducing healthcare costs to the insurer, which may reduce health insurance premium increases as a result of the reduction in healthcare costs for the group.

Pearls of WISDOM

Determining funding methods takes you into uncharted territory. EMS has typically used a cost-based pricing model, charging enough for services so that given the rate of collection, you will be able to at least cover your costs. For example, if your cost per transport is $400 and your collection net or net rate is 30%, you'd have to charge $1,334 to cover your cost of transport (400/0.30). Funding methods for MIH are totally different. Yes, you need to know your cost of delivering the service, but for the first time, you have the opportunity to be paid based on what the payer perceives as valuable. In almost every case that MedStar offered a price for an MIH service, it was discovered that the payer's perspective was cost avoidance, and they were more than willing to pay based on that premise. If your MIH program is going to save the payer $1,200 per patient enrolled, ask for a percentage of the savings versus a true cost-plus pricing model.

Are You READY?

- Conduct a meeting with various external stakeholders to discuss relevant metrics they would consider useful in measuring the outcome performance of an MIH program to determine possible funding opportunities.

- Complete a full analysis of your potential cost to deliver an MIH program based on:
  - Total cost to deliver

- Cost per patient contact
- Cost per patient enrolled

■ Read the Agency for Healthcare Research and Quality (AHRQ) report called *Trained Paramedics Provide Ongoing Support to Frequent 9-1-1 Callers, Reducing Use of Ambulance and Emergency Department Services* to see how they assign value at: http://www.innovations.ahrq.gov/content .aspx?id=3343

Summary

Developing and implementing an MIH program in many cases is like drawing on a blank canvas. You may have some ideas and concepts based on successes in other communities, but the final product is all up to the artist. The same is true of the funding models. As illustrated in this chapter, your funding model options are only limited by your imagination.

A few things to remember:

■ Follow the money!

■ Seek funding partners early, and have them help you design programs they might be willing to fund.

■ Remember there is no national standard for these models, so you have flexibility.

■ Be creative!

■ Price your services based on both the perceived value to the payer and the cost of delivering the service.

References

1. Department of Health and Human Services, Centers for Medicare & Medicaid Services. Instructions to accept and process all ambulance transportation healthcare common procedure coding system (HCPCS) codes. Available at: http://www.cms.gov/Outreach-and-Education/Medicare-Learning-Network-MLN/MLNMattersArticles/downloads/MM7489.pdf. Accessed June 26, 2014.

2. Office of the Inspector General. Provider compliance training: Take the initiative. Cultivate a culture of compliance with health care laws. Available at: https://oig.hhs.gov/compliance/provider-compliance-training/files/StarkandAKSChartHandout508.pdf. Accessed June 26, 2014.

9

Where Do You Go from Here?

At this point, you've probably considered many of the ideas presented in the book, and chances are you're ready to ignite change! Where do you start? It can seem overwhelming. The first step is always the hardest, but the most important. The greatest risk communities face given the rapid-fire changes occurring in the healthcare system is *paralysis by analysis*. Franklin Delano Roosevelt provided an appropriate quote for where you are right now: "There are many ways to move forward, but only one way to stand still."

It's time to move forward.

Use your accomplishment of finishing this book as a discussion starter. It may go like this:

You know, I just read this book on mobile integrated healthcare and believe many of the concepts being used in Ft. Worth, Wake County, western Pennsylvania, Eagle County, and Reno may have some real applicability to our community. What would you think about…?

Here's a checklist to get you started.

Organizational Readiness Assessment

✓ Medical director on board

✓ Chief/executive on board

✓ Labor/workforce on board

✓ City/county management on board

Community Assessment

✓ Local stakeholders

✓ Healthcare industry

✓ Regulatory industry

✓ Nongovernmental agencies

✓ Elected officials

✓ Peer EMS agencies

Convene Needs Assessment Forum with:

✓ Hospitals

✓ Skilled nursing

✓ Home health

✓ Hospice

✓ Community service agencies

✓ Payers

✓ Elected officials

Plan it!

✓ Start small (**Figure 9-1**)—a single project.

✓ Determine goals, success, and metrics.

✓ Determine training needed based on the project.

✓ Determine resource needs.

✓ Conduct training.

✓ Educate the community.

Do it!

✓ Implement a small-scale program.

- Limited number of patients

- Limited interventions

- Limited time frame

Study it!

✓ Did the plan work?

✓ What did you learn?

✓ What should you do differently?

✓ Do you need to make any changes?

Act on the review!

✓ Make changes.

✓ Refine the program or process.

✓ Add more services?

Repeat above

Mobile integrated healthcare is an innovative new frontier, and in many ways, by taking on the challenge of implementing this type of program, you're a trailblazer. It takes a commitment to leadership, innovation, and growth. Engagement is the key to success. How well are you communicating with people in your community and healthcare organizations? Are you establishing their trust, and are they responding positively to your ideas?

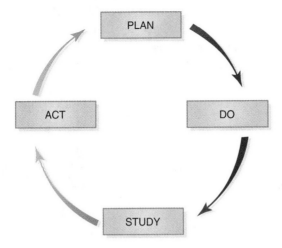

Figure 9-1 IHI model used as a framework to guide improvement developed by Associates in Process Improvement.

Data from: Langley GL, Nolan KM, Nolan TW, Norman CL, Provost LP. The improvement guide: a practical approach to enhancing organizational performance, ed 2. San Francisco, CA; Jossey-Bass; 2009

During implementation of an MIH program, there will be setbacks and obstacles; however, you can turn them into opportunities for learning and growth. If you're not making mistakes, you're not innovating. If you think you're doing everything perfectly, it's probably because you're not looking hard enough to find the things that you could be improving. Part of the learning process involves seeking feedback from your internal and external constituents and partners in the community you serve.

Part of your organizational readiness assessment is to ask yourself how easy is it for you to try something new. The culture must be prepared to innovate. Transformation requires change, openness, and a willingness to step out of your comfort zone and embrace change.

Start by adopting a mindset and culture of innovation internally. Make sure that your organization's leadership, both clinical and operational, is willing to try something new. Make the investment to convince your internal stakeholders that change is coming. They can either choose to be in the caboose, or to be in the engineer's seat.

MedStar has had the opportunity to meet with more than 100 different communities to discuss MIH services as a viable addition to improve patient care. The following are key points to remember during your discussions.

Core mission: The core mission is to provide healthcare to individuals who need help, to serve the community to make it a healthier place to live and work, and to make the most efficient use of the resources entrusted to us. MIH is the answer to achieving the core mission.

Home health: The role of MIH is to help patients navigate to the most appropriate sources of healthcare, not to replace healthcare services already available to them. If home health resources are available in the community and the patient qualifies for home health, those services should be used. There are, however, communities in rural areas in which home health is not available or patients who don't qualify for home health. The transitional time between the patient being referred to home health and the home health agency making the first visit may be a logical gap for you to fill.

Money: Share that many agencies are receiving ample payment not to transport patients to the hospital. And, there is more than likely already enough financial resources in the ambulance and healthcare industry to improve patient outcomes by reallocating dollars spent on services with evidence of limited value (ambulance transport) to other methods that bring the right patient to the right care, at the right time, in the right setting, and at the right cost.

The goal of every MIH program should be to help local communities and the country meet the Institute for Healthcare Improvement's Triple Aim:

- Improve patient care (including the experience of care).

- Improve population health.

- Reduce costs.

Delivering the right care at the right time to the right patient in the right setting is the wave of the future—EMS is perfectly positioned to have a dramatic impact on this care delivery transformation.

Results!

MedStar and other communities that have implemented effective MIH programs have seen incredible clinical, operational, and community relations results since the inception of the MIH program. Several key principles account for the successful program.

1. Identification of local community healthcare needs

2. Collaboration with the local healthcare system stakeholders to drive every aspect of the programs

3. Integration with, not replacement of, existing resources

4. Involvement of physician leaders who are committed to the program and patients

5. Starting small, with demonstration projects and short cycle testing to see what works

6. Not being afraid to make mistakes, learning from mistakes, and building the program from there

VOICES OF EXPERIENCE

I truly value the relationship HealthSouth Rehabilitation Hospital has with MedStar. Their level of expertise has been demonstrated consistently with the ability to identify patients with rehab potential. We've had the privilege to work with MedStar's elite medics, and their professionalism is unsurpassable. Collaborating with the team is beneficial not only to our patients but the community as a whole. HealthSouth is proud of the working relationship that we have and look forward to continuing community service together.

Keary Jones, MBA, BSN, RN
HealthSouth Rehabilitation Hospital
Fort Worth, TX

While the national debate on health care reform continues, EMS providers are in a key position to make the biggest difference in the healthcare system since the National Academy of Sciences in 1966 published the famous white paper *Accidental Death and Disability: The Neglected Disease of Modern Society,* which lead to the creation of modern EMS.

The ultimate decision now is yours. The healthcare environment is fundamentally changing. These changes will affect everything you do. You can choose to be part of the engineering team to design that change, or not. If you choose not to change the way you provide healthcare, another agency in your community will, with your stakeholders. What's your choice?

Pearls of WISDOM

Do not be afraid to fail! The only way to learn is to earn a few scars. At a recent board of director's retreat, one of MedStar's board members stated, "Scar tissue is wisdom." Thomas Edison has three famous quotes when it comes to invention and innovation. Try to live by these as you embark down the road of innovation:

"I have not failed. I've just found 10,000 ways that won't work."

"Our greatest weakness lies in giving up. The most certain way to succeed is always to try just one more time."

"Opportunity is missed by most people because it is dressed in overalls and looks like work."

MIH and Community Paramedicine Programs in the United States

Regional Emergency Medical Services Authority (REMSA), Reno, NV

Program Goals and Methods

- Create new patient care and referral pathways that ensure patients who have entered the 9-1-1 EMS system with urgent low-acuity medical conditions receive the safest and most appropriate levels of quality care.

- After hospital discharge, patients with conditions such as congestive heart failure will receive in-home follow-up care.

- The Nurse Health Line provides 24/7 assessment, clinical education, triage, and referral to health care and community services by way of a nonemergency nurse health line available to all Washoe County residents regardless of insurance status.

- Community health paramedics are specially trained to perform in-home delegated tasks to improve the transition of care from hospital to home, perform point-of-care lab tests, and improve patient adherence to the care plan.

- The Ambulance Transport Alternatives Program provides alternative pathways of care for 9-1-1 patients, including transport of psychiatric patients directly to the mental health hospital, transport of intoxicated patients directly to the detoxification center, and transport of 9-1-1 patients with low-acuity medical conditions to urgent care centers and clinics.

Outcomes

These programs will safely improve patient-centered care, reduce ambulance transports, reduce ED visits, reduce hospital readmissions, improve patient satisfaction, and reduce overall healthcare costs.

Program Funding

These programs received a 3-year, $9.5 million Health Care Innovation Award (HCIA) grant from the Centers for Medicare & Medicaid Innovation

Wake County EMS, Wake County, NC
Program Goals and Methods

The Advanced Paramedic Program is the EMS arm of the mobile integrated healthcare practice in Raleigh/Wake County, NC. The program works with Medicaid, hospital-based, mental health, primary care/medical home, and other public safety partners to ensure that patients receive time-appropriate care that matches their needs. In addition to providing "traditional" EMS care, alternative care (such as in-home treatment and transport to care facilities other than the ED) is provided for patients in the system. The following highlights three program goals:

- **Respond:** Advanced practice paramedics are scheduled to frequently be available to respond to high-acuity patients, particularly those in cardiac arrest. The outcome measure of interest is neurologically intact survival, which is reported to the Cardiac Arrest Registry to Enhance Survival (CARES) database as well as via local reporting with our hospital partners.

- **Reduce:** The goal of this program is to reduce unnecessary transports to the hospital emergency department. The Falls in Assisted-Living Facility Program is the most visible program in this area, whereby patients who experience a simple fall are evaluated by a specific protocol. If no emergency medical condition is xml:identified, the patient's primary care physician is contacted and follow-up within 18 hours in the assisted-living facility is arranged. This is a consent-based, institutional review board approved, ongoing prospective trial. The outcome of interest is the incidence of time-critical medical or trauma conditions.

- **Redirect:** The goal of this program is to offer transportation and treatment options in addition to transport and treatment in the hospital ED. The most visible program in this area involves patients with mental health and substance abuse issues. Patients with primary complaints in these areas are evaluated based on a set of protocols and, if they are found to be an appropriate candidate for redirection to a facility other than the ED, they are offered transport to a crisis center, mental health hospital, or faith-based detox facility. Measures of outcomes include subsequent referral to an ED for an emergency medical condition and ultimate outcome of the patient.

Outcomes

- **Respond:** In 2013, there was an overall patient survival of 14%, 90% of whom were neurologically intact. Patients with an initially shockable rhythm had an overall survival of 38%, with a 98% neurologically intact survival.

- **Reduce:** More than 150 patients have been evaluated (with the goal of evaluating 1,500 patients in order to validate the protocol); interim safety analysis is pending, but currently there are no known adverse outcomes related to the protocol.

- **Redirect:** Advanced practice paramedics provided the initial EMS response to 1,503 calls over a 1-year period:
  - Of the 1,503 patient encounters, 514 (34.2%) met diversion eligibility criteria, and 315 (61.2%) of those eligible agreed to be transported to WakeBrook instead of the local ED.
  - Only 4 (1.3%) patients transported to WakeBrook were referred back to the ED, none of whom subsequently required medical intervention.
  - Among the patients treated at WakeBrook, 199/315 patients (63.2%) were treated and discharged home with mental health follow-up. We estimate the program saved 2,448 ED bed hours and 100 hospitalizations and reduced costs of care by $500,000.

Program Funding
This project was self-funded.

Center for Emergency Medicine – Western Pennsylvania, Pittsburgh, PA
Program Goals and Methods

- Improve patient outcomes and experience of care.

- Reduce preventable ED visits and hospitalizations.
  - Primary focus—familiar faces and vulnerable patients

- Regional service delivery model with referrals from 45 EMS agencies and 15 hospitals in Allegheny County (Pittsburgh and surrounding communities)

- Complete psychosocial assessment by a community paramedic, who then serves as a patient navigator, patient advocate, and health coach to ensure patients become enrolled in applicable social service agencies

Outcomes

- Over 250 patients referred to program since its launch in September 2013.

- One patient had 29 EMS trips to the ED for uncontrolled hypoglycemia prior to enrollment in the program. Since enrollment, the patient has returned to the ED once for a problem with his fistula. Estimated savings of $21,000 in avoided EMS trips and ED costs was determined.

Program Funding

This program received a 2-year, $500,000 grant funded by very competitive integrated delivery systems.

Christian Hospital EMS, St. Louis, MO
Program Goals and Methods

- Improve population health.

- Improve patient outcomes and experience of care.

- Navigate nonmedical emergency patients from using EMS and ED.

- Reduce EMS and ED use for nonmedical emergencies.

- Decrease financial loss in ED and EMS for nonmedical emergencies.

- Ambulance and a specially trained paramedic responds to low-acuity calls.

- Patients are triaged and receive medical screening. If no medical emergency exists the patient is not transported to the hospital. The patient will be treated at home or an appointment with the health resource center or primary care physician is set up.

Outcomes

- Navigated 1,100 patients with nonmedical emergencies away from the ED

- Decreased EMS and ED volume by 11%

- Decreased EMS and ED use with this group 22% since February 2014

Program Funding

This program was awarded $100,000 grant from the hospital foundation. Contracts are pending with private payers and accountable care organizations.

Eagle County Paramedics, Eagle County, CO
Program Goals and Methods

- Ensure all patients have a medical home.

- Reduce rehospitalizations by 50%.

- Enhance injury prevention awareness to reduce potential costs associated with no prevention.

- Increase number of vaccinations given and public health visits.

- Single community paramedic designated to provide care to the rural community.

- Follow-up visits after hospital discharge

- Follow-up visits with primary care physician

- School-based health programs

- Injury prevention programs in the community

- Public health programs

- Social Services adult protection visits

- In-home lab services

- Starting a new mental health and substance abuse program with the county and hospital

Outcomes

- Community paramedic team was part of the hospital team that reduced readmissions over 76% in the local hospital in 2013

- Health care expenditure savings per patient visit was $1,279.

Program Funding
This program was self-funded.

North Memorial Medical Center, Minneapolis, MN
Program Goals and Methods
Sixteen community paramedics in three primary clinics in the North Minneapolis area:

- 12–14 patients per 12-hour shift

- Assigned patients by a clinic coordinator

- Primary care focused

- Patients need to have a care plan or be in a medical home.

- Medical home and care plan avoids duplication of service.

- Focus on patients with chronic disease with emphasis on patients with diabetes

- Assistance with wound management

- All lab work completed on site.

- Tracks frequent patient ED use with follow-up.

Outcomes
Outcomes continue to be tracked unofficially, with outcomes subjectively thought to be very positive. Work at the state level to develop a common data base to show the positive results of using a community paramedic. Data should be available soon. The current healthcare delivery system

medical assistance demo project with 6,000 enrollees has shown an overall reduction in per-member, per-month cost of medical assistance. With the reduction there is a shared savings payment to the healthcare system from managed care and state fee-for-service.

Program Funding

- Community paramedics were integrated into a Medicare shared savings accountable care organization program with 10,000 enrollees.

- Community paramedics primarily target the medical assistance population in a state healthcare delivery system demo with 6,000 enrollees.

- Medical assistance covers eligible community paramedic services at the rate of $60 an hour if the patient is in a primary care plan or assigned to a medical home.

San Diego Fire-Rescue Department & Rural/Metro Ambulance, San Diego, CA

Program Goals and Methods

- Preserve public safety and acute care response resources through strategic initiatives for vulnerable populations at the systemic and client level.

- Reduce 9-1-1 use in high-utilizer group (HUG) patients using specially trained paramedics who proactively and reactively surveil the 9-1-1 system and intervene to provide care coordination.

  - Proactive interventions are initiated in response to first responder electronic referrals as well as predictive data algorithms that focus on classification of vulnerabilities (such as in-home fall risks, substance abuse, and mental illness).

  - Reactive interventions are initiated when a patient is electronically ranked in a weekly top 10 position for 9-1-1 use.

  - The program uses data mining technology to surveil, predict, xml:identify, and alert practitioner on patients of interest in near real-time.

Outcomes

A pilot study of 51 individuals with 10 or more EMS transports within 12 months demonstrated resource access program success. The San Diego EMS Resource Access Program is a paramedic-based surveillance and case management system that intercepts high EMS users.

- EMS transports declined 37.6%, from 736 to 459, resulting in a 32.1% decrease in EMS charges from $689,743 to $468,394.

- EMS task time and mileage decreased by 39.8% and 47.5%, respectively, accounting for 262 hours and 1,940 miles.

- ED encounters at the one participating hospital declined from 199 visits to 143 (28.1%), which correlated with a decrease in charges from $413,410 to $360,779 (12.7%).

- Inpatient admissions declined from 33 to 30 (9.1%), and inpatient charges declined from $687,306 to $646,881 (5.9%). Hospital length of stay was reduced from 122 to 88 days (27.9%).

- Across all services, total charges declined by $314,306.

Program Funding
This project was funded by Rural/Metro Ambulance.

Mesa Fire & Medical Department, Mesa, AZ
Program Goals and Methods

- Implementation of priority dispatch from an all-hazards advanced life support response to utilization of two 2-person community paramedic units and two 2-person community care response units, in which one of those units has a nurse practitioner and the other a behavioral health specialist provided through local partnerships.
    - Each of these units has a captain/firefighter/paramedic on the response apparatus.

- Reduce the number of behavioral health 9-1-1 calls by deployment of a 2-person behavioral health prevention unit.

- Reduce preventable 9-1-1 low-acuity calls by 30% through proactive visits of high utilizers of the EMS system to enhance education and management of chronic diseases with referral to primary care providers.

- Reduce unnecessary ambulance transports of low-acuity medical and traumatically injured 9-1-1 callers to EDs with appropriate care and referral to the patient's primary care medical home.

- Reduce ambulance transports of behavioral health and substance abuse 9-1-1 callers to EDs by providing on-scene crisis intervention and appropriate transport to behavioral health/substance abuse facilities for definitive care.

- Reduce hospital readmissions of cardiac patients who have undergone an intervention.

- Reduce hospital readmissions by bridging the gap in coverage of patients referred to the Mesa Fire & Medical Department as they await authorization of home health services as requested by the discharging hospital.

- Decrease 9-1-1 response times by 25% to advanced life support calls, fire response, and others requiring a four-person firefighter response.

- Achieve 80% cost recovery for services rendered by the community care response units.

- Develop quality care metrics to enhance patient assessments and care provided to better measure the delivered services to better comply with Triple Aim goals.

Outcomes

- 11-second (5%) reduction in 9-1-1 response times

- Over 300% reduction in costs associated with all-hazard response

- $3.4 million savings to the healthcare systems with the City of Mesa, AZ

- Responded to a total of over 3,000 low-acuity calls (approximately 25% of local demand)
  - 1,508 community paramedic responses with fire paramedic and fire EMT (approximately 10% of local demand)
  - 1,250 community care responses with fire paramedic and nurse practitioner (approximately 25% of local demand)
  - 242 behavioral health responses with fire paramedic and behavioral health specialist (approximately 40% of local demand)

Program Funding

- Initial pilot in 2008 was funded by a $100,000 Arizona Department of Health Services grant.

- Presently self-funded through the Mesa Fire & Medical Department budget ($600,000/year)

- Cost recovery is currently under development.

- All programs are in jeopardy due to lack of ability to implement billing and cost recovery.

Methodist Hospital and Fire Departments in St. Louis Park, Edina, Minneapolis, Richfield, Eden Prairie, Minnetonka, and Hopkins, MN

- Program Goals and Methods: Follow-up after hospital discharge.

- Outcomes: None yet (in development)

- Program Funding: Pending (discussing $50–100 per patient contact)

Green Bay Fire and Bellin Health, Green Bay, WI

- Program Goals and Methods: Follow-up after hospital discharge.

- Outcomes: None yet (in development)

- Program Funding: $50 for one safe transition patient contact at home.

Additional Resources

In addition to the resources included in the book chapters, the following links and reading materials will help you more fully understand the concept of mobile integrated healthcare and community paramedicine.

Overview and updates on data metrics for MIH programs at MedStar Mobile Healthcare
www.medstar911.org/community-health-program

NAEMT dedicated website with catalogs of documents, databases, and general information on MIH/CP
http://www.naemt.org/MIH-CP/MIH-CP.aspx

National Association of State EMS Official's research and report on MIH/CP programs
https://www.nasemso.org/Projects/MobileIntegratedHealth/

National Association of Emergency Medical Services Physician's link to the joint position statement on MIH/CP
http://www.naemsp.org/Documents/PRESS%20RELEASE%20NAEMT-Vision-News%2002-06-14.pdf

Integrated Healthcare Delivery magazine—full of information on the spectrum of care across the continuum
http://ihdelivery.com/

North Central EMS Institute link for MIH/CP
www.communityparamedic.org/

International Roundtable on Community Paramedicine—U.S. and international models and information on MIH/CP
www.ircp.info/

HRSA community paramedicine evaluation tool
www.hrsa.gov/ruralhealth/pdf/paramedicevaltool.pdf

State of Nebraska's overview of community paramedicine
www.dhhs.ne.gov/Documents/CommunityParamedicineReport.pdf

Article in *New York Times* on MIH/CP
www.nytimes.com/2011/09/19/us/community-paramedics-seek-to-prevent-emergencies-too.html

Community paramedicine report from the University of California – Davis
https://www.ucdmc.ucdavis.edu/iphi/publications/reports/commparamed.html

American Medical Association position paper published in February 2013 *Journal of the American Medical Association* on the realignment of EMS payments to improve care and reduce costs
http://jama.jamanetwork.com/article.aspx?articleid=1653531

Article in *Health Affairs* detailing the economic benefit of realigning EMS payments
http://content.healthaffairs.org/content/32/12/2142.abstract

American Nurses Association position statement on community paramedicine
http://www.nursingworld.org/MainMenuCategories/ThePracticeofProfessionalNursing/NursingStandards/ANAPrinciples/EssentialPrinciples-UtilizationCommunityParamedics.pdf

Modern Healthcare Magazine article on MIH
http://info.modernhealthcare.com/rs/crain/images/Medtronic_Download_12-9.pdf

Hennepin Technical College community paramedic training information
https://www.hennepintech.edu/customizedtraining/cts/44#&panel1-1

North Memorial Health Care summary of 1st year of community paramedicine
https://www.northmemorial.com/communityparamedic

Numerous podcasts on MIH/CP
http://www.mediccast.com/blog/tag/mobile-integrated-healthcare/

EMS leadership podcast on the NAEMT MIH summit in Washington, DC
http://www.emsleadership.com/?tag=mobile-integrated-healthcare

Index

Note: Page numbers followed by *f* and *t* refer to figure and table, respectively.